Magnet
Therapy

Magnet Therapy

*The Gentle and
Effective Way to
Balance Body
Systems*

Ghanshyam Singh Birla
and
Colette Hemlin

Healing Arts Press
Rochester, Vermont

Healing Arts Press
One Park Street
Rochester, Vermont 05767
www.InnerTraditions.com

Healing Arts Press is a division of Inner Traditions International

*Note to the reader: This book is intended as an informational guide. The remedies, approaches,
and techniques described herein are meant to supplement, and not to be a substitute for,
professional medical care or treatment. They should not be used to treat a serious ailment
without prior consultation with a qualified health care professional.*

Library of Congress Cataloging-in-Publication Data

Birla, Ghanshyam Singh, 1941–
Magnet therapy : the gentle and effective way to balance body systems
/ Ghanshyam Singh Birla and Colette Hemlin.
p.   cm.
ISBN 0-89281-841-7 (alk. paper)
1. Magnetotherapy—Popular works.   2. Self-care, Health.   I. Hemlin, Colette.
II. Title.
RM893.B55   1999   99-37558
615.8'45—dc21   CIP

Printed and bound in Canada

10 9 8 7 6 5 4 3 2

Text design and layout by Priscilla Baker
Original illustrations by Sophie Bisaillon and Colette Hemlin
This book was typeset in New Baskerville

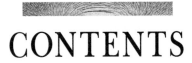

CONTENTS

To the memory of the late Dr. Benoytosh Bhattacharyya, a pioneer in the field of magnet therapy, and to his beloved son, Dr. A. K. Bhattacharya, who follows in his father's footsteps promoting the advancement of alternative medicine for the service of humanity.

ACKNOWLEDGMENTS

Ages ago, the enlightened Indian sage Kanada (the atom-eater), recognized the magical effects of attraction and repulsion among a handful of seemingly simple stones and posited that a natural energy field must be responsible for this inherent quality. Kanada's conclusions and his further theories developed ultimately into one of the six major systems of the Indian philosophy called *Vaisesika* (from the Sanskrit root *visesus,* meaning scientific knowledge).

My heart goes out to that brilliant expounder Kanada, whose enlightened curiosity and willingness to explore the power and potency of magnets, continues to provide inspiration in the emerging field of magnet therapy.

I am also thankful to many of our modern researchers and scientists, and to all pioneers of magnetic therapy, whose open-minded receptivity has brought a new dimension to this age-old therapy with the purpose of healing humanity at large. I owe a special debt of gratitude to the late Albert Roy Davis.

As a personal growth consultant, for over thirty years now, I use a variety of Vedic sciences, such as Jyotish, Samudrik Shastra, meditation with mantras, yoga, and various Ayurvedic healing techniques, to help my students and clients find balance and self-understanding in their own lives. Several years ago, I became interested in the power of magnets as healing tools. This book is the result of my queries.

I would like to thank many who encouraged me in my explorations of the subject. Firstly, Dr. A. K. Bhattacharya of the Naihati Homeopathic Clinic in West Bengal, whose groundbreaking writings and subsequent friendship have always been a beacon to my efforts.

As well, Dr. P. K. Biswas, vice-chancellor of the University of Alternative Medicine, Drs. Usha and K. K. Kapoor, Dr. Suman Motilal Shah of Calcutta, India, and Dr. Donald Lorimer have all provided, and continue to provide, inspiration to me on my magnetic quests.

I am especially grateful to my coauthor Colette Hemlin, who enthusiastically agreed to embark upon the task of putting all my notes and observations into this form you are holding in your hands now. Her energy and ever vigilant curiosity for additional research have added a profound depth to the material.

As for our magnificent editing staff, Virginia (Nazneen) Wallis, Johanne Riopel, Agnes Jacob, Victoria Ridout and Jacinthe Côté, all deserve a heartfelt thanks for their perspicacity in translating, typing, and proofreading the manuscript.

My deepest thanks to my loving colleagues, astrologer-palmists, massage therapists, reflexologists, Kathleen Keogh, Marie-Claire Sauvé, Peter Keogh, Guylaine Vallée, Elyise Trépanier, Grace Macklin, Denise Parisé, Chandan Rugenius, and Rémi Riverin, who objectively implemented magnet tests and passed along their research results to create the foundation of this work. Special thanks to Heather Flockhart, who has coordinated for nearly two decades our magnetic research department at the Palmistry Center.

Eternal gratitude to my beloved wife Chanchala, my daughter Rekha, and sons Keero and Abhishekananda, who have always encouraged my efforts to promote self-understanding through the Vedic sciences.

Finally I am eternally grateful to my Paramguru Sri Sri Swami Yukteswarji, whose precious book *The Holy Science* continues to serve as a great inspiration to explore the principles of universal magnetism from the macrocosmic to the microcosmic level in all human beings; all living magnets striving for perfect equilibrium, peace and joy, within and without.

Ghanshyam Singh Birla

FOREWORD

It was indeed a great pleasure and honor to receive a request from my very good friend Dr. Ghanshyam Singh Birla to write a foreword for his new book *Magnet Therapy*. We have been acquainted with each other for more than two decades and I knew him to be an able astrologer and palmist but this book gives indications of his versatile genius. In spite of our academic acquaintance, we first met each other in person in 1996 during the centenary celebrations for my father Dr. Benoytosh Bhattacharyya. Dr. Birla came to attend the functions with his family and students and spent a few days with us. During this time I learned of his deep interest in the use of magnets and the result was this book. Apart from palmistry and astrology which he teaches at his Palmistry Center and National Research Institute in Canada, Dr. Birla is also very much interested in gem therapy, teletherapy, and so forth. Someday we may find a new book written by him on one of these subjects.

Some time back Dr. Birla sent me his manuscript for the new book on magnets but due to very heavy work pressure I could not write the foreword immediately or send my views on the book, for which the book was delayed. I beg to be excused by the author and also the readers for delaying the publication of such a wonderful book.

The book is very well written and contains a mine of information on the subject of magnets that is not available in other books on this subject. To understand the subject it is very important to understand the history of its origin. *Magnet Therapy* covers this historical aspect with a thoroughness that will interest readers.

The second chapter deals with different types of magnets, natural and artificial. Dr. Birla details the industrial uses of these permanent magnets and describes the different types for ease of understanding.

The third chapter looks at the properties of magnets and the different types of magnets. This chapter provides an academic background on the subject and will help readers understand the relative values and strengths of magnets.

The fourth chapter, Biomagnetism, describes experiments done with magnets on plants and animals by various researchers in different parts of the world. It also describes the effects of magnetism on human beings. This is a most important chapter that will give the reader insight into the effects of magnets on different human systems such as the nervous system, circulatory system, endocrine system, and so forth. This chapter will enable the reader to put magnets to practical use.

The fifth chapter provides a guide to the treatment of different ailments of the human body. By studying this chapter carefully, beginners at magnet therapy can learn specific techniques for relieving ailments.

The sixth chapter deals with the effect of magnetized water on plants, animals, and humans. Readers who want to test the effectiveness of magnets should try this simple experiment with magnetized water. It will convince everyone of the efficacy of this therapy. One should remember that "the proof of the pudding is in the eating."

The seventh chapter provides case reports of patients treated with magnet therapy that will help readers to try their hands at this novel system.

In conclusion, alternative systems of medicine are gaining recognition from the general public due to the inefficacy of the modern system and the mounting costs of treatment. Magnet therapy is very easy, inexpensive, and also very effective in many cases. In my experience I have found magnets particularly effective for relieving any kind of pain or inflammation. If magnets did no more than relieve pain, that would be enough of a valuable service. Every system has its limitations; if readers use magnets with the full understanding of their usefulness provided in *Magnet Therapy,* I am sure nobody will be disillusioned.

I compliment Dr. Ghanshyam Singh Birla for writing such a wonderful book and I strongly recommend that everyone not only read it but also put it into practice. I wish Dr. Birla success in all future ventures.

Dr. A. K. Bhattacharya
Director, Naihati Homeopathy and Magnetotherapy Clinic
West Bengal, India
President, World Teletherapy Organization

INTRODUCTION

Health is a state of balance that everyone would like to acquire and maintain. In recent years, people have become more careful about their eating habits, and many try to include exercise in their daily routine. Some have also taken up holistic health–promoting yoga, meditation, mantras, tai chi, and other such disciplines.

In many cases, these habits are enough to maintain an optimal state of health. Yet sometimes illness strikes just the same. People often feel helpless when they are ill and in pain, and in North America their first impulse is to turn to conventional medical treatments. But when conventional medicine is not effective, as with chronic illness, or is too invasive, people often begin to look for other solutions. More and more people are turning to alternative treatments like Ayurvedic medicine, acupuncture, or homeopathy. In fact, it is estimated that in 1990 Americans spent ten billion dollars on alternative therapies and medicine.

Magnet therapy is an alternative treatment that has been gaining ground in recent years. There are many reports of successful applications throughout Europe, Asia, and North America. In Holland, patients suffering from chronic conditions like Parkinson's disease have experienced notable improvement. In Japan, double-blind tests have demonstrated a 90 percent success rate in the treatment of stiff necks and shoulders, lumbago, rheumatism, and other common conditions. Over ten thousand people reported significant pain relief after average-strength (590-gauss) permanent magnets were applied over a period of four days or less. It is estimated that in the early 1990s hundreds of thousands of Americans were using magnets for therapeutic purposes; the number of people using magnet therapy throughout the world today is almost one hundred million.

However, despite these impressive numbers, magnet therapy is still rejected by most traditional doctors or simply ignored as an alternative treatment. Even though the therapeutic value of magnetism has been demonstrated and observed for years, many people are not aware of this effective treatment. In light of this, we feel it is important to provide a clear and simple explanation of magnet therapy so that more people have the opportunity to experience its benefits.

Magnet therapy is closely related to biomagnetism—a branch of biology that studies the effects of magnetism on living beings—as well as magnetism and electromagnetism. This book will discuss the origins of these three disciplines, all of which have long histories of study and use. Very ancient texts, like the Vedas of India, indicate that magnetic phenomena and effects were recognized and recorded from the earliest times. Later texts, like those of the Greek physician Galen from the second century A.D., describe the use of magnets for healing purposes. However, the tools necessary for the accurate and in-depth study of biomagnetic phenomena have only recently become available. In this sense, biomagnetism is a relatively new science.

In the nineteenth century, magnet therapy was applied tentatively and advanced by trial and error. Over time practitioners kept records of what worked and what didn't. But it is only recently that these observations were explained scientifically. As a result, we now know the precautionary measures to use with magnet therapy, and we are now able to promote magnet therapy as a very safe and effective treatment when used correctly.

As indicated earlier, many experiments with magnet therapy have been conducted all over the world, and in this book we will report on the results of those experiments. We have also experimented for a number of years at our own institute,* using magnets to reduce pain and balance metabolic functioning. Our observations have convinced us of the extensive health benefits of magnetism.

In this book we will attempt to explain, in simple terms, what magnetism is: what we know about it, how it works, how it can be used to improve health, and what precautionary measures should be taken when using magnets. We hope to demonstrate that you do not need to be a physicist, biologist, or doctor to understand and benefit from magnet therapy.

We believe that magnet therapy is the perfect method to create balance in your life. If you follow the instructions given in this book, you will soon see notable improvements in your physical, mental, and emotional health. We do not claim that you will never need a doctor again, but you can expect to achieve more control over your health. You will be surprised how quickly and easily a properly used magnet, or some magnetized water, can bring balance back into your life; or how you can make a headache disappear without medication, or relieve insomnia without sleeping pills.

What more is there to say? Instead of accepting all the little annoying ills of life, or just waiting for them to go away, you can use magnet therapy to restore balance. The marvelous power of magnets can help maintain good health, increase your energy level, and strengthen your immune system. We believe that you will be pleasantly surprised by the results. However, we wish to emphasize that it is very important that you follow the safety instructions at the beginning of chapter 5.

IMPORTANT NOTE

When applying the principles of biomagnetism, it is very important to use the right polarity (for reasons we will explain later).

---

*The National Research Institute for Self-Understanding (The Palmistry Center) was founded by Ghanshyam Singh Birla in 1972 to promote self-understanding through the ancient Vedic arts and sciences of palmistry, astrology, and related disciplines, such as mantra chanting, gem therapy, magnet therapy, and Ayurvedic healing principles. The institute was expanded in 1998 with the opening of Village Lac Dumouchel, a 300-acre retreat and health center.

However, we wish to point out that there is no consensus about the designation of the magnetic poles. "North pole" and "south pole" mean different things to different people. Therefore, magnets are not always marked "north" and "south" in the same manner.

When a permanent magnet is left to hang freely, it spins for a short time and then stops on the north-south axis of the earth. One of its faces—always the same one—points to the north, and the other points to the south. In 1269, Pierre de Maricourt was the first person to differentiate the two poles of a magnet. He decided to call "north" the pole that points to the geographic north pole and "south" the pole that points to the geographic south pole. Later, it became clear that opposite poles attract and same-type poles repel each other. Therefore, it would be more logical to call "north" the pole of a magnet pointing to the geographic south and to call "south" the pole pointing to the geographic north.

According to most physics books, the magnetic south pole is located in the northern hemisphere, in the Canadian Arctic, because induction lines come together there; and the magnetic north pole is located in the southern hemisphere, in Antarctica, because induction lines emerge from there. However, an Energy Mines and Resources Canada document submitted to the Geomagnetism Division of the Earth Physics Branch states that the magnetic north pole is located near the geographic north pole, specifically slightly north of Bathurst Island, and that it is there that induction lines come together. Several biomagnetism specialists (Albert Roy Davis, Walter Rawls, etc.) share the same view: They liken the north pole to a negative charge and the south pole to a positive charge.

Some magnet manufacturers identify the poles in the same way de Maricourt did, but others use the more logical method. This can be problematic when buying a magnet because you don't know on what basis the manufacturer has identified the poles. This confusion about the terms "north pole" and "south pole" can interfere with the understanding and development of biomagnetism.

However, it is not our intention to explore this question. We merely want to point out that there is no consensus on the correct way of naming the poles, and therefore no one method is

4

correct or incorrect. For the sake of clarity, in this book the term "north pole" will designate the place where induction lines come together, and the term "south pole" identifies the place where they emerge. We also associate the poles with the characteristics listed in table 1.

TABLE 1

Magnetic North Pole	Magnetic South Pole
Induction lines converge	Induction lines reemerge
Negative	Positive
Presently located at the geographic north pole	Presently located at the geographic south pole

Chapter One

HISTORY

THE HISTORY OF BIOMAGNETISM

Although biomagnetism has only recently begun to be recognized by Western science and medicine, its origins are in fact very old. The effect of magnetic stone on iron has been known since ancient times, and many cultures have believed in the ability of magnets to cure certain illnesses. For centuries the people of India, China, and the eastern Mediterranean basin, as well as Australian aborigines and native Africans, were all familiar with the use of magnets. And certain paintings suggest that the high priests of ancient Egypt used magnets in some of their religious ceremonies.

The therapeutic use of magnetism dates back to very early times. In his book *De Simplicium Medicamentorum Temperamentis Ac Facultatibus*, the Greek physician Galen noted that magnetism was being used for its purgative powers around 200 B.C. Around A.D. 1000, a Persian physician named Ali Abbas was using magnetism to treat "spasms" and "gout." In the sixteenth century, Paracelsus, an innovative Swiss physician, claimed to cure "hernias, gout, and jaundice" through the use of magnets. Around the same time, Ambroise Paré, a French surgeon who authored several medical books and later became known as the father of modern surgery, provided instruction on how to heal open wounds and injuries with finely powdered magnetite mixed with honey.* However, although these and other individuals understood the effect of magnetic fields on living beings, biomagnetism was not a widely recognized discipline in past centuries.

THE HISTORY OF MAGNETISM

To understand the history of modern biomagnetism, it is necessary to examine the earlier history of magnetism and electromagnetism. Electromagnetism is a relatively new field that emerged only a few hundred years ago, but the knowledge of magnetism goes back to ancient times.

According to legend, a shepherd named Magnes discovered a mineral that attracted the nails of his sandals (or the end of his cane in some versions) as he crossed Mount Ida in Asia Minor some twenty-five hundred years ago. Today, that mineral is known as magnetite. Other sources claim that the word "magnetism" comes from Magnesia, a city in ancient Asia Minor where the stone could be found. At some point it was observed that when a magnet is left free to spin, it always comes to rest in the same position. We don't know exactly when this discovery was made, except for the fact that in 1269 Pierre de Maricourt differentiated the two poles. During the twelfth century A.D. this characteristic of magnets was being used in navigation by the Arabs, the Vikings, and the Europeans. The use of some form of magnetic compass was also commonly in use by the Chinese around A.D. 100.

However, detailed experiments and observations about the properties of magnetism were not documented until much later. Magnets are mentioned in several documents written before the thirteenth century, but the "broken magnet" experiment, which demonstrates that a magnet is actually composed of many smaller magnets, was not known until A.D. 1269. At that time, European

---

*The therapeutic properties of honey are described very clearly by Dr. H. C. A. Vogel in *Le petit docteur* (Geneva: Jean-René Fleming, 1991).

seamen were aware that the magnetic needle of a compass did not always point exactly to the geographic north, a phenomenon recorded by the Chinese of the Tang dynasty almost seven centuries earlier. Although the exact nature of magnetism was not yet known, around 1550 the Flemish cartographer G. Mercator, who created the first map of the world, succeeded in solving, more or less, the problem of locating on a map the geographic north indicated by the magnetic needle. And in 1600, William Gilbert, the official court physician of Queen Elizabeth I, published his famous work *De Magnete,* which summarizes all that was known and believed about magnetism in the Elizabethan age and attests to the use of magnets in the treatment of illness.

It was not until about two hundred years later in the eighteenth century that the principles of magnetism began to be better understood. At that time, a renewed interest in the study of magnetism was developing throughout Europe among doctors, chemists, and especially physicists. German physician Franz Anton Mesmer was the first in a long line of scientists to claim that the properties of the magnet offered a cure for all illness. When he came to Paris from Vienna in 1778, his doctrine, known as mesmerism, briefly aroused great interest due to some well-publicized cures. Mesmer believed that all living beings are subject to the influence of a "magnetic fluid" that can be collected and rechanneled by "passes" and manipulation. A little later, in 1791, during his famous experiment conducted on frogs to study the effects of electricity on muscles and nerves, Italian physicist Luigi Galvani discovered what he believed to be the "animal magnetism" espoused by Mesmer. However, the spontaneous contractions observed in the experiment were not in fact caused by animal magnetism but rather by electrochemical phenomena.

The modern term "biomagnetism" refers to the study of the sensitivity and reaction of living organisms to the earth's magnetic field and to artificial magnetic fields having similar intensities. The term is relatively recent and has replaced Mesmer's term "animal magnetism."

In 1778, the Dutch physicist Anton Brugmans discovered

diamagnetism, a characteristic of those elements (including mercury, silver, and zinc) that are slightly repulsed by magnets. In the eighteenth and early nineteenth centuries, French physicist and engineer Charles-Augustin de Coulomb went on to establish the experimental and theoretical basis of magnetism and electrostatics. He was the first to make quantitative measurements of electric attraction and repulsion and to formulate a law governing these phenomena.

Another contribution to the field of magnetism came from Denmark. In 1820, Danish physicist Hans Christian Ørsted conducted his famous experiment demonstrating that a magnetic needle is deviated by an electric current, which suggested that magnetism could be described in terms of currents, even if those currents could not be observed by the human eye. This observation became the foundation of the field of electromagnetism.

THE BIRTH OF ELECTROMAGNETISM

Until the nineteenth century, electricity and magnetism were treated as two different branches of physics even though many important connections were known to exist between them. After Ørsted's discovery of electrical currents in 1820, the gifted French scientist, mathematician, and physicist André-Marie Ampère took only a few days to formulate the theory of electromagnetism, and a new field was born. Ampère studied the influence that currents and magnets have on each other and theorized that magnetism is based on the existence of particular currents. He also invented the galvanometer, the first electric telegraph system, and the electromagnet. In the same year as Ørsted's discovery, French scientist Dominique François Arago demonstrated that an iron bar could be magnetized if it was placed in a solenoid through which an electric current runs. Until that time, the only permanent magnets were those found in nature, and Arago's discovery led to the manufacture of artificial magnets.

The nineteenth century was the golden era of physics. Throughout Europe, discoveries followed one another at an amazing pace.

The English scientist William Sturgeon built the first electromagnet in 1825, using a horseshoe-shaped iron bar coated with varnish (which acted as an insulating agent) and wrapped in bare electric wire. However, the resulting electromagnet was not very strong and could lift only a few grams.

In 1831, a few years after the discovery of electromagnetism, British physicist and chemist Michael Faraday discovered the principle of electromagnetic induction. Electromagnetic induction is the production of electric current in a circuit by variations in the flux of magnetic induction to which the circuit is subjected; most modern electric generators and transformers depend on it. Faraday, who carefully recorded his more than sixteen thousand experiments and research projects, went on to become the father of several other new branches in the field of magnetism, including electromagnetism and magnetic force lines. A year after Faraday's discovery of electromagnetic induction, American physicist Joseph Henry made the same discovery more than two thousand kilometers away. Faraday was the first to publish his findings and therefore the discovery was attributed to him, but the unit measuring electrical inductance in the International System of Units, henry or H, was named after Joseph Henry.

German astronomer, mathematician, and physicist Carl Friedrich Gauss, who made numerous discoveries in mathematics as well as in astronomy, also chose magnetism as his main field of interest. In 1839 he formulated the mathematical theory of magnetism and invented the magnetometer. His name was given to the magnetic induction unit in the centimeter-gram-second measurement system.

The Scottish physicist James Clerk Maxwell is known mostly for his contribution to the kinetic theory of gases and the discovery of magnetostriction (the phenomenon of substances changing in volume when placed in a magnetic field). However, he is first and foremost the author of the electromagnetic theory of light (1865), for which he devised the general equations of the electromagnetic field. In fact, Maxwell's theory combines electric and magnetic phenomena, and his equations play the same role in electromagnetism as

Newton's principles and the law of universal gravitation do in the field of mechanics.

English physicist Oliver Heaviside and Dutch scientists H. A. Lorentz and Heinrich Hertz later clarified Maxwell's theory, which caused the electromagnetism branch of physics to grow considerably. Hertz proved the existence of "Maxwellian waves," now called short radio-electric waves. The inventor Guglielmo Marconi worked on the practical application of these waves and conducted the first radio transmission in 1896. In 1898 Danish engineer Valdemar Poulsen invented magnetically recorded sound, which many of us could not imagine being without! Many more applications of magnetism soon followed. Today, magnets and the practical application of magnetism are present in almost every aspect of our lives, from the magnetic levitation systems used in transportation and the magnetic resonance devices used in medicine to audio and video systems, personal computers, calculators, and doorbells.

Around 1895, the French physicist Pierre Curie established a clear distinction between paramagnetism, a property of those elements that acquire a weak magnetic charge of the same type as the field they are placed in, and diamagnetism, a property of those elements that acquire a weak magnetic charge opposite to that of the induction field. Based on an observation William Gilbert had made three hundred years earlier, Curie identified a rise in temperature as the characteristic that signaled a change from ferromagnetism, a property of those elements that acquire a strong magnetic charge of the same type as that of the induction field, to paramagnetism, and he discovered that each substance has its own critical temperature point beyond which it loses its ferromagnetic property. The critical temperature at which this change takes place is now known as the Curie point.

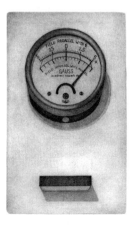

Fig. 1. Magnetometer

BIOMAGNETISM

Scientific interest in magnetism had almost disappeared by the early twentieth century. However, while most doctors and physicists concentrated their efforts on other areas of study, throughout the world a number of researchers continued the study of magnetism. They usually worked discreetly, as their work was often not taken seriously and was sometimes discredited by their colleagues. Nonetheless, they persisted in their endeavors.

In the mid-1930s, various studies and research reports dealing with magnets and the applications of magnetism to health problems started to emerge. For example, between 1935 and 1937, Dr. William Campbell of Cambridge University studied the physical effects of magnetic fields on rodents and other small animals. In Germany, Dr. H. Bingenheimer attempted to establish the effects of electromagnetic energy on living organisms in the hope of using electromagnetism to stimulate physical development. A little later, between 1956 and 1971, Dr. N. S. Hanoka of the University of Israel studied the effect of magnetic fields on the reduction of infection and the treatment of injuries. Researchers in other countries were involved with various other related studies, some of which confirmed what others had discovered before them.

Today efforts are ongoing to effectively apply magnetic properties to physiology. There have been many experiments and studies conducted in the United States, Germany, Russia, and other countries that have begun to establish the effects of magnetic fields on living organisms, and those experiments continue. However, even though these studies employ rigorous research methods, medical sectarianism often discounts therapies based on magnetism, as it does other alternative treatments and therapies. The development of biomagnetism has also been hindered by a lack of necessary equipment. Instruments able to measure very low-intensity magnetic fields, such as those found in the human body, have only recently become available.

In fact, it was not until 1911 that the German physician Heike

Kamerlingh Onnes established the theory of superconductivity, a discovery that finally made it possible to manufacture the tools and instruments necessary to measure biomagnetic signals of very low intensity, such as those in the human body and heart. (Superconductivity is a characteristic of certain metals whose electrical resistance disappears almost completely at temperatures below a specific threshold, usually very low, around 5°K, or -268°C. The resistance of supraconductors is practically nil; a current flowing in a supraconductor circuit can last for weeks without decreasing, even though the circuit has no generator. But as soon as the temperature is raised slightly above the threshold the current quickly falls to zero.) Thus, the birth of biomagnetism can only be said to have taken place in 1962, when G. H. Baule and R. McFee succeeded in taking the first magnetocardiogram.

Another highlight in the study of magnetism is the discovery of the elementary magnetic moment, or magneton, made in 1921 by Otto Stern, a German-born American physicist. As a result of Stern's work, we now know the magnetic properties of atoms. Later, in 1954, American chemist Linus C. Pauling was awarded the Nobel Prize in chemistry for his discovery of the magnetic properties of hemoglobin. This was a crucial discovery, and we now know that iron is not only involved in transporting the oxygen in hemoglobin, but also plays an important role in cell metabolism. All these discoveries have given us a better understanding of the effects and applications of magnetic and electric fields and have also contributed to the development of various magnetic resonance equipment now used in the field of medicine.

The study of biomagnetism continues to expand. The first International Conference on Biomagnetism took place in Boston in 1976. This conference was more a forum for discussion than a formal conference. Subsequent conferences saw a large number of presentations on subjects such as neuromagnetism, cardiomagnetism, and other practical applications of biomagnetism. In 1991, the eighth International Congress on Biomagnetism, held in Münster, Germany, was attended by four hundred participants from over thirty countries, featured more than 240 presentations on various aspects of biomagnetism, and produced a total of 142 papers, which were eventually published in a nine-hundred-page book entitled *Biomagnetism: Clinical Aspects.** By that time, improved data gathering in multiple areas made it possible to include a much greater number of clinical studies, which became the subject of the most recent conference.

At first, research in the field of biomagnetism was conducted only in physical-science or engineering laboratories, simply because the equipment was not available elsewhere. When the Superconductivity Quantum Interference Device (SQUID) system became generally available around 1971, research was extended to include the biological sciences. Since the early 1990s, this new field of knowledge is even being applied in clinical settings. However, powerful biomagnetic equipment is expensive, and less effective biomagnetic systems are only used in clinical environments when nothing else can replace them. When other less expensive systems are able to produce the same results, they can be used instead of the current biomagnetic devices. Researchers are in the process of trying to develop limited systems that cover the patient's head or chest only, which would be less expensive alternatives to those that cover the whole body.

It is clear that the improvement of existing biomagnetic systems, as well as the reduction of their considerable production costs, will be necessary before this science can flourish in the medical realm. The development of data interpretation models is also a priority. Once data have been gathered they must be compared to a consistent standard in order to identify exceptions. The challenge in biomagnetic research is to create strategies that lead to reliable conclusions, which can then be used to make accurate diagnoses and suggest effective treatments. At the current level of research and practice, biomagnetism is still a field restricted to a small number of practitioners.

---

*M. Moke, S. N. Erné, Y. C. Okada, and G. L. Romani, eds., *Biomagnetism: Clinical Aspects,* proceedings of the eighth International Conference on Biomagnetism held in August 1991 in Münster, Germany (Münster, 1992).

Information sources for the general public are also limited. Although several scientists have shown an interest in the application of biomagnetism to medical practice, very few have written works accessible to the general reader. The exceptions are B. Bhattacharyya and his son A. K. Bhattacharya, Albert Roy Davis, Dhanlal Gala, Holger Hanneman, Larry Johnson, Buryl Payne, Walter C. Rawls, Ralph U. Sierra, G. W. de la Warr, and George J. Washnis, who have all written books that are appropriate for the layperson.

The study of magnetism has an important place in the culture of India, which is why much of the significant research on biomagnetism comes from there. The ancient Vedas speak of the polarity present in each human being and in each atom, and Indian doctors commonly use magnetism in their practice. Earlier this century Dr. Benoytosh Bhattacharyya conducted important research in the therapeutic power of magnets and gems and wrote several books on the subject. A. K. Bhattacharya, his son, has continued his father's work and gone on to study the effects of magnetism on biological systems (plants, animals, and human beings). He has also researched the clinical applications of magnetism in cases where traditional medicine has proved to be ineffective, and like his father he has written many important works on the subject, including several on biomagnetism.

Dr. Kyoichi Nakagawa, director of the Isuzu Hospital in Tokyo, spent more than twenty years researching the effects of magnetism on living beings and discovered that a shortage of magnetism could be the cause of certain medical disorders in a growing number of people. He found that although the symptoms of those disorders are not characteristic of what he calls Magnetic Field Deficiency Syndrome, they respond only to the application of magnetic fields. We will discuss this phenomenon in greater detail later.

Dr. Albert Roy Davis (1915-1984), an American researcher born in Canada, studied the two different energy fields characterizing magnetism, and it is because of this work that we know the effect of the south pole is different from the effect of the north pole on a magnet. Dr. Davis was a member of the American Association for the Advancement of Science and the New York Academy of Sciences, and scientists in both India and Japan have acknowledged his important contribution to the advancement of biomagnetism.

This history of biomagnetism, including the earlier history of magnetism and electromagnetism, shows how old the knowledge and study of this important field are. It also identifies some of the factors that have delayed the emergence of biomagnetism as an effective, established, and widespread means of diagnosis and treatment. However, before exploring the subject further, it is necessary to examine the physical properties of magnetism and of magnets, the instruments that are employed in the application of biomagnetism and are reputed to have such amazing powers. The best place to start is the origin and composition of magnets.

Chapter Two

TYPES OF MAGNETS AND THEIR PRODUCTION

There are essentially two types of magnetism: the natural magnetic energy of the earth, or geomagnetism, which has a very low but constant intensity and operates in a gigantic field; and the magnetism produced by magnets and electromagnets, the intensity of which is usually stronger but more limited.

GEOMAGNETISM

Despite all that has been discovered about magnetism in the last two hundred years, the origin of geomagnetism is still uncertain. Some physicists propose that there is a giant permanent magnet in the center of the earth, a magnetic mass or electric current that is responsible for the earth's magnetic field. Others theorize that the earth's magnetic field actually originates at a great distance from the earth. Still others suggest that this magnetic field is created by the ionization of the layers of air surrounding the earth. It is likely that all three hypotheses are partly true.

The earth can be considered a giant permanent magnet whose

origin is both internal and external, and the same can be said of other planets in the solar system. Scientists have long suspected the existence of a magnetic field around Mars, and that theory has now been proven by the Mars Global Surveyor space probe. Although the field around Mars has a polarity similar to that of the earth, its intensity is only one eight-hundredth of the earth's field (it is not known whether that intensity level has remained constant throughout the existence of the planet). It appears that Jupiter and Saturn also have magnetic fields.

INTERNALLY GENERATED MAGNETISM

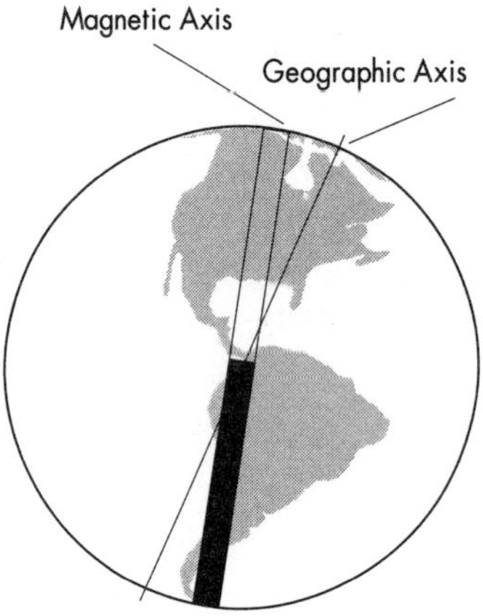

Fig. 2. The Earth: A Giant Magnet

Part of the earth's magnetic field is generated internally. Geophysicists believe that most of the earth's iron is concentrated in the planet's core and therefore is highly conductive. They also believe that the earth has a solid internal core and an external core in a state of fusion. Although no one has explored the depths of the earth that far, we do know that its magnetic field is produced by many electric currents of various origins contained in the earth's core, such as the currents produced by the interaction of local magnetic fields and the rotation of the earth, and Foucault currents produced by convection in the liquid core of the earth. The measurable magnetic field on the earth's surface is about 0.5 gauss, and that field extends up to 64,000 km from the surface of the planet, forming a zone known as the magnetosphere. The earth's magnetic field exerts continuous action on all living organisms, both plant and animal.

Based on the study of seismic waves and below-surface temperatures and the recording and analysis of magnetic phenomena, scientists are able to provide the following description of the interior of the earth: It is believed that the inner core is composed mostly of iron, as well as other metals, and has a radius of about 1,280 km and a temperature that reaches 5,000°C. The outer core is believed to be composed of rock in a state of fusion and is estimated to be about 2,000 km thick. The earth's mantle has a possible thickness of about 2,800 km, whereas the earth's crust is believed to measure only 40 km.

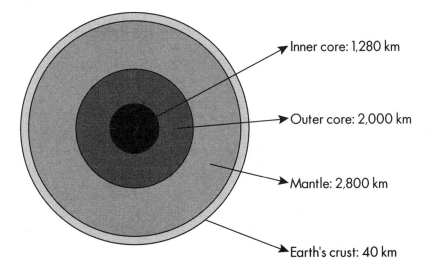

Fig. 3. Cross Section of the Earth

The measurable characteristics of the earth's magnetic field include intensity (about 0.5 gauss at present), declination, inclination, and the horizontal component of induction. Magnetic maps provide these measurements, which vary according to the location at which the measurements are taken. There can also be local irregularities caused by the geological particularities of the underlayer.

The earth is like a giant magnet with two magnetic poles, but those poles should not be confused with the earth's geographic poles. In fact, since the time of Christopher Columbus navigators

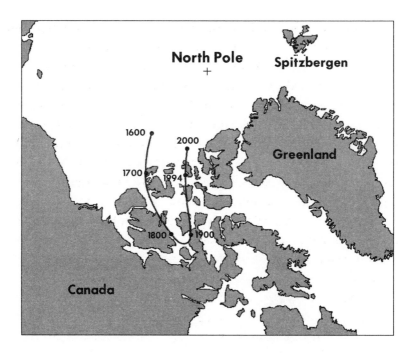

Fig. 4. Movement of the Magnetic North Pole

have observed that a magnetic compass does not indicate the true geographic north but is deviated east or west depending on the observer's position. The earth's magnetic poles are located near its geographic poles, and their positions are said to shift continuously. Between 1900 and 1970, the magnetic north pole moved approximately 720 km toward the geographic north, from a location close to Boothia Peninsula to slightly north of Bathurst Island. Recently the movement of the pole has accelerated; it now moves approximately 15 km per year. In 1994, the magnetic north pole was positioned at 78°3' north latitude and 104° west longitude, near Noice Peninsula, slightly southwest of Ellef Ringnes Island.

In the past scientists believed the earth was composed of stable elements. However, we now know the earth is actually a dynamic body made up of moving and variable elements. The earth's main geomagnetic field is subject to slow variations, which are neither uniform nor constant. In other words, the intensity of the geomagnetic field can increase in one region of the globe and decrease irregularly in another. These variations originate from the interior of the earth and may not occur for long periods.

A science called paleomagnetism studies magnetic remanence in rocks, especially those in the Canadian Shield, whose formations are among the oldest on the surface of the planet. This science researches phenomena occurring hundreds of millions of years ago. Experts in the field have established that in the last seventy million years the earth's magnetic field has reversed itself abruptly more than a hundred times. This means that there are times when the magnetic north pole has been located nearer the geographic south pole. It has even been proven that in the last four million years the earth's magnetic axis has completely reversed direction at least nine times.

According to the Earth Physics Branch at Energy Mines and Resources Canada, Earth's magnetic north pole is currently located near the geographic north pole. However, some researchers are convinced that it is actually located near the geographic south pole. They base this assertion on the sixteenth-century work of William Gilbert, which sheds some light on this controversy.

EXTERNALLY GENERATED MAGNETISM

Earth's magnetic field, whose source is mainly internal, is magnified by the variations in magnetic fields caused by electric currents in the ionosphere. It is also affected by the continuous energy of the sun, or solar wind.

It is generally agreed that sunspots are formed by the very high-intensity magnetic fields generated deep inside the sun, and we know that some sunspots can be eight times larger than the earth. Solar energy emanates from the sun, causing electrified gas eruptions that spin and produce a magnetic field whose influence is felt on the earth. The appearance of sunspots varies in space and time, but solar activity has an approximate twenty-two-year cycle. Some scientists have postulated an eleven-year cycle, but most believe that sunspots actually move from north to south for eleven years and south to north for another eleven years.

At the height of solar activity, the number of sunspots appearing on the surface of the sun can reach between 150 and 200 in a single month, and it is said that the conditions for radio transmission are excellent during these periods. The constant flow of energy from the sun (solar wind) causes variations in the electric currents of the ionosphere but does not seem to affect the earth's magnetic field, except in high-latitude regions like Canada.

It is inside auroral zones that the most violent magnetic storms are formed, as well as the aurora borealis (the colored reflection of electric energy in the ionosphere, also known as northern lights). These zones are also characterized by the greatest radio transmission interference. The geomagnetic field in the Arctic and Antarctic regions is complex as well, which causes problems in the preparation of magnetic maps used by land surveyors, navigators, and geologists. Because of the frequent magnetic variations in these regions, new maps have to be prepared every five years, carry a date, and include the annual changes foreseen for each of the coordinates.

The earth's magnetism (about 0.5 gauss) is much weaker than that of the sun (about 25 to 50 gauss). Yet the earth exerts a constant magnetic influence that can be seen in the following experiments: If you allow a magnet to spin freely (hanging or balanced on an axis), it will turn in a particular direction (north-south axis), and this direction will never change. And if you place an iron bar horizontally in a north-south axis for a certain period, the end pointing south will acquire north polarity.

There can be no doubt that the earth is a giant permanent magnet whose energy has significant effects on all living beings, be they plants, animals, or humans. But before we examine the nature of those effects, we need to define what magnets are and identify their composition and properties.

NATURAL PERMANENT MAGNETS

The first magnets noticed and used by humans were natural magnets of volcanic origin. When lava emerges from a volcano, propulsed outward from inside the earth, it cools gradually, locking in the earth's magnetism. When the lava has completely cooled, it forms a stone that has absorbed a certain amount of the magnetic energy at the center of the earth. However, it is the iron content of the volcanic stone that will determine its magnetic power. The natural iron oxide Fe_3O_4, a black ferromagnetic ore that has a high iron content, is known as iron magnetite or magnetic stone. Fragments of this natural magnetic stone are available, but their magnetic force is usually limited and varies from one stone to another.

ARTIFICIAL PERMANENT MAGNETS

Today, natural magnets are rare and infrequently used. They have been replaced by artificial magnets, which are of variable composition but usually made mostly of iron. Such magnets have been known in Europe since the twelfth century. In the eleventh century, the Chinese discovered that iron could be magnetized by heating it until it is red-hot and then cooling it while it is kept in a north-south axis. Permanent artificial magnets are composed of different elements, producing magnets with different properties that can be used for different purposes. The main advantage of artificial magnets is that they can be given shapes that suit their required use. They can also quickly acquire a much stronger magnetization than that of natural magnets.

Artificial magnets can be produced by two methods. One method is to rub a magnet on a ferromagnetic substance, in one direction only, thus conferring a weak magnetic charge to the substance. The disadvantage of this method is the low intensity of the new magnet.

The more frequent method used to produce artificial magnets creates a weak or strong magnetization in only seconds. Ferromagnetic material is placed inside a solenoid (a spool of

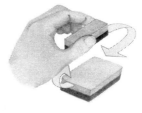

Fig. 5. Magnetization by Friction

electric wire twisted into a spiral around a bobbin in the form of a cylinder and fed by a continuous current). Depending on the material used, this method produces either a temporary magnetization (with iron, for example) or a remanent magnetization (with tempered steel, which is an alloy of iron and carbon), which remains after the magnetic field has been removed. Iron is known for its greater retention and is easily magnetized; however, it has low coercibility (resistance to demagnetization) and thus loses its magnetization easily. Therefore, steel is the preferred material for producing permanent magnets, and iron is considered the best element for producing electromagnets.

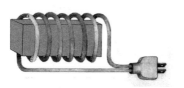

*Fig. 6. Magnetization
with a Solenoid*

ARTIFICIAL METALLIC MAGNETS

Artificial magnets are either metallic or synthetic. Most metallic magnets are a mixture of aluminum, nickel, iron, and cobalt, which together compose an alloy known as alnico. Over time, methods have been developed to produce magnets that are more stable and less expensive to produce. Table 2 shows the different types of alnico alloys that can be used to produce metallic magnets. In each case, iron is the main component because it is inexpensive.

Some metallic magnets are made mostly of neodymium, a rare

TABLE 2: CHEMICAL COMPOSITION OF ALNICO

Metal	Percentage of Alnico	Percentage of Alnico II	Percentage of Alnico III	Percentage of Alnico IV
Aluminum	18	10	12	8
Nickel	––	20	24	14
Cobalt	12	12	––	24
Copper	6	6	3	3
Iron	64	52	61	51

Source: R. S. Bansal and H. L. Bansal, *Magneto Therapy Self-Help Book*

element discovered in 1885. Neodymium magnets are more expensive than alnico magnets, but they are more powerful. They are used mostly in the treatment of cancer and are not necessary for home use. They are also less readily available than alnico magnets.

ARTIFICIAL SYNTHETIC MAGNETS

Some magnets are made of synthetic materials, such as ceramic or graphite magnets. The advantages of synthetic magnets are a high coercibility and the ability to maintain magnetism for long periods. These magnets show greater stability in the face of demagnetization fields and temperature changes and usually weigh up to 60 percent less than metallic magnets. They are also less expensive to produce, need little care or special maintenance, and are more shock resistant than metallic magnets.

Because of these characteristics, synthetic magnets are used mostly in the fields of communications (speakers, microphones), electricity (dynamos, small engines, toys, instruments), electronics (calculators, computers), and transportation (car radios, dynamos, tape players, motor scooters) and in many other common products (doorbells, automatic doors, magnetic games, etc.).

ELECTROMAGNETS

All permanent magnets, whether natural or artificial, metallic or synthetic, have the same basic properties. However, electromagnets are a completely different type of magnet. When a continuous electric current passes through a solenoid, a more or less uniform magnetic field is produced inside the instrument. This is the method used to produce electromagnets. When the current inside the solenoid is stopped, the magnetic field effect also ceases immediately. Because the main advantage of electromagnets is the ability to quickly activate and deactivate the magnetic field effect, electromagnets are made of iron, which has greater retention and lower coercibility.

Because electromagnets create an electric field in addition to a magnetic field, they are used primarily in scientific laboratories. Electromagnets produce a different effect than permanent magnets; the magnetic field is more uniform than that produced by a permanent magnet, and the field ceases to exist as soon as the electric current is stopped. Unfortunately, in addition to producing an electric field that is sometimes undesirable, this method is not able to produce a particular desired polarity. For that reason, this book will not explore electromagnets and electromagnetism further.

Chapter Three

PROPERTIES OF MAGNETS

Now that we have looked at the origins and composition of magnets, we will explore their physical properties—characteristics that apply to all magnets, regardless of their origin, size, composition, or strength. However, it is necessary to explain some basic terms of magnetism before we examine those properties in detail.

Magnetic field: A magnet (or an electric wire with current passing through it) is surrounded by a field that attracts objects. This is called the magnetic field.

Magnetic induction: The basic vectorial dimension used to describe the magnetic field is known as magnetic induction and is described in terms of length and direction. Graphically, magnetic induction is represented by induction lines (just as force lines represent an electric field).

Induction lines: These are drawn so that the number of lines per the surface area perpendicular to them is proportional to the intensity of the field. This means that tightly grouped lines represent a strong field, whereas more sparsely placed lines represent a weak field.

Magnetic strength: The number of lines per given surface area determines the strength of a magnet. For instance, a 1,000-gauss magnet is stronger than a 500-gauss magnet and can attract more iron. (Please note that in physics, the terms "strength" and "power" are not synonymous. However, for our purposes it is not necessary to explain the sometimes complex difference between these two concepts.)

Flux: The flow of magnetic energy that circulates is known as the flux of the magnet.

PHYSICAL PROPERTIES OF MAGNETS

You have no doubt observed that the attraction-and-repulsion phenomenon can take place at a certain distance from a magnet. As indicated above, the zone in which a magnet produces its effect is called the magnetic field. We will discuss this field later in more detail. However, for now, we will examine the main magnetic effects existing in this field.

MAGNETIC PERMEABILITY

Have you ever noticed that a magnet sticks to the refrigerator door but not to the door of the microwave oven? This is because the doors are made of different materials. In the study of magnetism there are four categories of materials, which are classified according to the degree to which they are able to attract a magnet. The importance of each category varies.

Experiment: Using a rather strong magnet, try to move small objects made of different materials—for instance, a pencil (watch for the metal band), an eraser, a paper clip, silver jewelry, copper wire, wool thread, a candle, cooking salt, coins of different sizes, and so forth. According to your observations, divide these objects into two groups: materials that react to the magnet (Group A) and those that do not react (Group B). Then see if the results of your experiment reflect the categorizations made below.

FERROMAGNETIC MATERIALS

The first category of materials comprises elements that react strongly to magnetic fields (Group A in your experiment). These materials are called ferromagnetic. All of the materials in this category are metals or alloys, are magnetized in the direction of the magnetic field, and are the only elements that acquire a strong magnetic charge that persists even outside the magnetic field. Magnetic induction lines pass through these materials easily.

Ferromagnetism is not the property of a single atom, but a characteristic of the interaction of adjacent atoms. In other words, the fact that some of the atoms of a substance follow the direction of the magnetic field does not make the substance ferromagnetic. When ferromagnetic elements are placed in a magnetic field, all the atoms near the magnet are moved in the same direction (see figure 7). But these materials have uneven susceptibility and permeability, which are dependent on the induction field.

Elements in the ferromagnetic category of materials include iron, nickel, cobalt, and various alloys. These substances are very sensitive to excessive temperature increases. Beyond the Curie point (1,043°K for iron), interaction between adjacent atoms stops and the substance becomes paramagnetic (the third category of materials, discussed below).

Ferrimagnetic Materials

A subcategory of ferromagnetic materials, ferrimagnetic materials comprise materials that have remarkable magnetic properties as well as great resistance. Ferrimagnetic substances have two types of magnetic atoms: Some move in the direction of the magnetic field and others move in the opposite direction. Interaction among these different atoms produces a medium magnetization in the direction of the induction field (see figure 7).

Ferrimagnetic materials are used mainly in high frequency transformers, for example, electronic equipment and computer memories. These materials also lose their characteristics when heated beyond a certain temperature.

ANTIFERROMAGNETIC MATERIALS

The second category comprises some of those materials that show little reaction to magnetic fields (Group B in your experiment). Antiferromagnetic substances are so named because the adjacent atoms of these materials point in opposite directions, which cancels the magnetic effect; their external magnetism is so weak as to be almost nonexistent. Heated beyond a certain temperature, called the Néel point, these substances also become paramagnetic.

PARAMAGNETIC MATERIALS

The materials belonging to the third category are called paramagnetic. They are also magnetized in the direction of the magnetic field, but they acquire a weak charge (see figure 7). The elements in this category include oxygen, platinum, sodium, aluminum, chrome, manganese, copper, and potassium. Certain elements of the human body also belong in this category, such as blood, muscles, and nervous system tissue. However, the slight magnetic reaction of these materials is difficult to observe unless a very powerful magnet is used. (This is why you will have placed some paramagnetic materials, like copper wire and aluminum paper, in the "nonreactive" Group B.)

DIAMAGNETIC MATERIALS

The last category comprises diamagnetic elements. These materials are magnetized in the direction opposite to the induction field but acquire a very weak charge. Consequently, they are slightly repelled by a magnet (see figure 7). Mercury, silver, copper, lead, and zinc are only a few of the many elements in this category.

DIRECTION OF INDUCTION FIELD

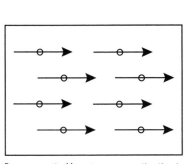

Ferromagnetic: Very strong magnetization in the direction of the induction field; iron, nickel, cobalt, alloys, and so on.

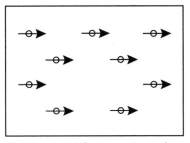

Paramagnetic: Weak magnetization in the direction of the induction field; oxygen, aluminum, copper, blood, muscles, and so on.

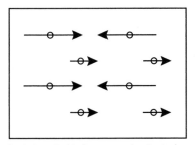

Ferrimagnetic: Medium magnetization in the direction of the induction field; bivalent metal-based ferrites (iron, manganese, cobalt, nickel), and iron alloys.

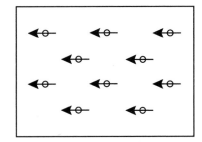

Diamagnetic: Very weak magnet-ization in the direction opposite to the induction field; repelled by magnets; mercury, silver, zinc, and so on.

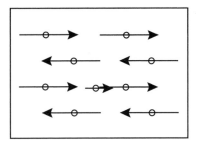

Fig. 7. Classification of elements based on their reaction to magnetism.

Antiferromagnetic: Very weak magnetization in the direction of the induction field; MnO_2.

HOW MAGNETISM WORKS

Physicists believe that each atom of an iron bar can be a magnet. Usually, atoms in an iron bar (or any other material) are grouped into "zones," regions in which the alignment of atoms is perfect. Each magnetic zone has a north and a south pole. These zones are located randomly in the iron bar when magnetic induction is weak. Magnetization consists of a parallel positioning of these zones, with the north pole of one zone facing the south pole of the one next to it (see figure 8). The north pole of a zone is then neutralized by the south pole of the adjacent zone, except at the two extremities of the iron bar.

DIRECTION OF INDUCTION FIELD

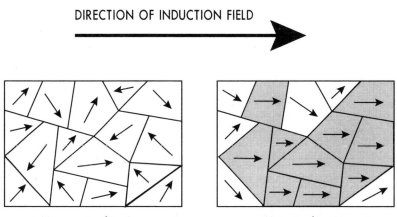

Nonmagnetized Iron Bar   Magnetized Iron Bar

Fig. 8. Distribution of Zones in an Iron Bar

Each extremity, then, has several south-pole or north-pole zones that are not neutralized. This is why only the extremities of a magnetized iron bar demonstrate magnetic effect. When magnetization takes place, the zones lying in the direction of the magnetic field cover a larger area than those lying in the opposite direction. Ultimately, when all the zones of the object are oriented in the direction of the magnetic field, the substance has reached its magnetic saturation level, and the magnet has exerted its greatest force.

MAGNETS ALIGN WITH THE NORTH-SOUTH AXIS OF THE EARTH

Experiment: Attach a magnet to a string and suspend it from a door frame or any other place from which it can hang freely. Observe the magnet for a few minutes, then repeat the experiment several times. What do you notice?

If a magnet is suspended at its middle, it will spin until it reaches a position of balance that is always constant. One of its ends (always the same pole of the magnet) will turn toward the north geographical pole. If the poles of the magnet are identified correctly, you will see that the south pole faces the north geographical pole. This characteristic helps in identifying the poles of magnets, as we will see later in this chapter. This same characteristic is the one that allows a compass to function, except that in a compass the magnetic needle is poised on a point instead of suspended.

EACH MAGNET HAS TWO POLES

A magnet has two poles, which are identified as north and south. A permanent magnet cannot have a north or south pole only. Some authors refer to magnets as being bipolar, meaning "having two poles." When a magnet is broken into two pieces, it produces two smaller magnets, each one having a north and south pole. This is easy to observe: If you accidentally drop a magnet, it will break into uneven pieces, and you can easily determine that each piece has two poles. The two poles of a permanent magnet are inseparable, and even the smallest particle of a magnet retains this property. The first recorded experiment demonstrating this

Fig. 9. Each Section of a Magnet Has Two Poles

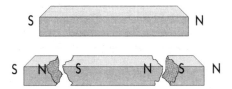

characteristic of magnets was conducted in 1269 and is known as the broken magnet experiment.

ATTRACTION AND REPULSION:
THE TWO EFFECTS OF MAGNETIC STRENGTH

Experiment: Bring two magnets close together. One of two things will happen: They will either attract each other or they will repel each other. Repeat the experiment several times, changing the position of the magnets. If the poles are marked accurately on the magnets, you will see that the ends with opposite polarities attract, and that same-type poles repel each other. (If the poles on the magnets are not indicated, refer to "How to Identify the Poles of a Magnet" on page 45 to learn two simple methods for identifying the po-larities.)

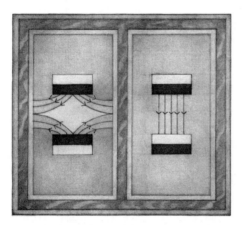

Fig. 10. Attraction/Repulsion: The Two Effects Produced by Magnetic Strength

This experiment demonstrates that the north pole of one magnet and the south pole of another are irresistibly attracted to each other. In contrast, the north pole of one and the north pole of another always repel each other, and the same is true of the south poles. Attraction and repulsion are the two manifestations of magnetic strength.

TWO EXTREMITIES OF A MAGNET
ATTRACT MOST STRONGLY

You will notice that the sides of very flat or long magnets attract very weakly. In other words, a magnet will attract nails at its north and south pole, but not much in the middle. As we explained earlier, this is because of the zones, which are all oriented in the same direction. Technically it is possible to isolate the poles of a magnet, even though they are actually inseparable. It can be done if we use only one end of a flat or a long magnet. However, in a horseshoe magnet the open end has both polarities very close to each other, and it is very hard to separate them.

If a nail is brought close to the end of a magnet, be it the north pole or the south pole, the nail will be attracted to the magnet indiscriminately. This is because the zones of the nail are polarized by the magnet according to the pole that is closest to the nail. If the nail is brought close to the north pole, the zones of the nail will be polarized in the direction of the magnetic field, and the south-pole points of the nail will automatically place them-

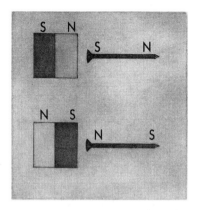

Fig. 11. Both Ends of a Magnet Attract Iron

selves near the magnet. The nail is sometimes magnetized strongly enough to attract other smaller nails, but not for very long. If immediately afterward the same nail is placed next to the south pole of the magnet, the polarity of the nail's different zones will reverse.

STRENGTH OF MAGNETS

The strength of a permanent magnet depends on several factors: its composition (each material having its own maximum value), the method of magnetization (rubbed in one direction with a magnet or electrically magnetized), the duration of magnetization, and the intensity of the current used. Remember that strong magnetic fields are graphically represented by lines that are close together and weaker fields are represented by lines farther apart.

Iron is easily magnetized, but it reaches its saturation level quickly. Therefore another material must be used to produce very strong magnets. Certain rare metals, such as neodymium, have a higher saturation level and can produce stronger magnets. However, such magnets are very expensive to produce.

If a strong magnetic field is required, electromagnets are often more convenient than permanent magnets. However, with an electromagnet the magnetic field ceases to exist as soon as the current is stopped, and unlike with permanent magnets it is impossible to isolate a single pole. There is also the problem of the effects created by electric fields, in addition to the magnetic field. Therefore, electromagnets should not be used without appropriate training and knowledge.

Magnetic strength is measured with a magnetometer and is usually expressed in gauss. The gauss is the unit of magnetic field intensity produced by a magnetic pole and measured at a distance of 1 cm from this pole. The oersted is the unit that measures magnetic field intensity in a vacuum. Because these measurements are about the same in air (gauss) and in a vacuum (oersted), these units can be used interchangeably. In other words, when the magnetic field is measured in air, either unit can be used. However, for the sake of simplicity, we will use gauss as the unit of magnetic intensity.

For each permanent magnet, strength varies depending on where on the magnet it is measured. If the greatest measurement obtained at a distance of 1 cm from the surface of a magnet is 300 gauss, the magnet is said to have an intensity of 300 gauss. When the measurement of a magnet is taken at its surface, we speak of surface measurement gauss. Magnetic induction is not evenly distributed on the surface of a magnet, and the magnetic field of a magnet is never as regular as drawings show it to be.

The strength of a magnet decreases as the distance from which the measurement is taken is increased; the greater the distance, the lower the intensity, and the magnetic effect diminishes quickly. Try this experiment with a magnet and a paper clip: As you move the clip farther from the magnet, there is a point when the magnetic effect is no longer felt. The distance at which this happens depends on the strength and shape of the magnet.

If we superpose two magnets of equal strength, we are not doubling the force of the magnetic field; the field will be increased only slightly. For example, if we take two 300-gauss (on the surface) magnets and place them on top of each other, the magnetic field produced will have a force of about 330 gauss on the surface—an increase of only 10 percent. If several equal-strength magnets are superposed, the maximum increase that can be obtained is about 35 percent. So there is no point in trying to obtain a 3,000-gauss field by using ten 300-gauss magnets. The maximum force that can be obtained in this way is 400 gauss on the surface.

If the magnets are placed in a checkerboard pattern, with alternating poles following each other, the surface measurement of the field—where the magnets intersect—will be only slightly higher than the strength of each magnet. In contrast, if the measurement is taken 1 cm away from the surface, the field will be weaker, because both poles are being felt.

CONSERVATION OF MAGNETISM (RETENTION)

The shape of a magnet seems to have an impact on its strength. Long magnets retain their magnetic charge longer than short ones. This is because, proportionally, the surface area that can become demagnetized is smaller for long magnets. Horseshoe magnets keep their charge even longer because they create a virtually closed circuit, and magnets with a hole maintain their charge longer still.

When a magnet is heated, beaten with a hammer, or twisted, its charge decreases because of a partial interruption of molecule alignment. A magnet that has not been optimally magnetized also tends to lose its magnetic charge with time. But whatever the cause of demagnetization, magnets can always be remagnetized. However, it is preferable to avoid accidental demagnetization when the magnet is not in use by keeping the two poles of the magnet tied together with a piece of soft iron, called a keeper. This serves to close the magnetic field and prevent loss almost completely.

MAGNETIC FIELD

As indicated, the area around a magnet is called the magnetic field, and this area is represented by induction lines. These lines are parallel to the magnet; they go in at one end and come out at the other, and they have no real beginning or end. As we move farther from the ends of the magnet, the lines become more spaced out. We know that magnetic effect can be felt from a distance in the air, but it is also true that magnetism can go through water, paper, fabric, and several other materials. When the magnet is strong enough (2,000 gauss or more), its effect can even be felt through a person's hand. By holding a magnet in the palm of your hand, you can move small metal objects (clips or pins) on a table without touching them. If the magnet is strong enough, you can even lift the object.

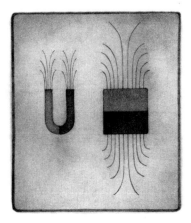

Fig. 12. Influence of the Shape of the Magnet on the Magnetic Field

Most magnets are said to be "open systems" because their north and south poles point in opposite directions. Horseshoe or U-shaped magnets are said to be "closed systems" because their north and south poles point in the same direction. A horseshoe magnet has a limited magnetic field because its magnetic effect operates in one direction only. In the case of open systems, the magnetic field is unlimited, at least theoretically, meaning that at a given distance from the magnet the attraction exerted is stronger than it would be in the case of a closed system of equal strength. Therefore, the magnetic field is infinite in principle, although beyond a certain distance the strength of any magnet is hardly perceptible and difficult to measure.

Of course, the greater the distance from the magnet, the more its strength is reduced; and this happens very quickly. It has also been observed that when two magnets are of equal strength, the magnetic force of the one with a greater surface area will be felt at a greater distance. For example, if we take two 500-gauss flat magnets of the same thickness, the first with 4 cm² of surface area (Magnet A) and the second with 9 cm² of surface area (Magnet B),

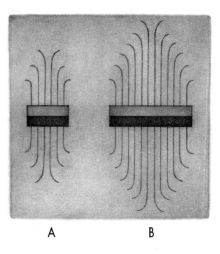

A   B

Fig. 13. Influence of a Magnet's Surface on the Magnetic Field

as shown in figure 13, the magnetic field of Magnet B will operate over a greater distance than that of Magnet A because the induction lines will not disperse as quickly. This is why magnets with a greater surface area are preferred in magnet therapy: They have farther-reaching magnetic fields and allow for greater penetration of induction lines.

MAGNETIC FIELD OF PERMANENT MAGNETS

The magnetic field produced by a permanent magnet is fixed but irregular. If we measure the force of the field at the surface of the magnet with a magnetometer, the measurements vary slightly as we move the instrument. This is why the strength of a magnet is given as the highest value recorded on the surface or 1 cm away.

MAGNETIC FIELD OF ELECTROMAGNETS

When electricity is passed through a spool of electric wire surrounding a metal (iron or steel) core, a very strong and effective magnet is produced. Each layer of wire on the spool has many magnetic induction lines, which are sometimes very powerful. When the current passes through the wire, the wire becomes heated, producing increased resistance to electricity. This causes either a slight decrease in the magnetic lines or an increase of magnetic strength, depending on the material of the electromagnet. Thus, vibrations produced by electromagnets are not as constant as those produced by permanent magnets. However, it is possible to regulate the frequency of the current, that is, the number of pulsations. It is also possible to vary magnetic intensity by controlling the current. But it is impossible to isolate a specific pole on an electromagnet, as can be done with permanent magnets.

MAGNETIC DISTRIBUTION

Certain theories about magnetism have been confirmed, whereas others have been discarded and replaced as a result of more advanced research. The theory concerning the nature of magnetic induction has developed over time, and today most scientists agree that energy flows from one pole of a magnet to the other, with induction lines coming out at one pole and going in at the other in a curved movement. The movement of induction lines was conceptualized by observing the configuration of iron filings on a glass plate lying on a straight magnet. Schoolbooks still teach this concept, which originated in 1936. Figure 14 is a classic representation.

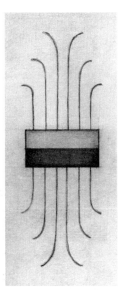

Fig. 14. Traditional Concept of Magnetic Distribution

Scientist Albert Roy Davis was convinced that this traditional concept is incorrect because it does not take into account the fact that each particle of iron filings entering the magnetic field itself becomes a magnet whose field affects adjacent particles. Laboratory experiments led him to believe that magnetism is distributed in the form of a circle in the center of the magnet, where the direction of the current is reversed. In other words, the trajectory of magnetic induction lines is shaped like a figure

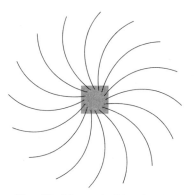

Fig. 15. Magnetic Distribution as Vortex, According to Dr. Davis

eight. Induction lines coming from the south pole form a vortex, a kind of swirl moving clockwise, that is, turning right. Lines entering the north pole form a vortex moving counterclockwise, that is, to the left. This direction is inverted at the center point of the magnet, and at that exact point the magnetic field is nil. All permanent magnets have in their exact center an invisible line that has no north or south pole attributes. Dr. Davis called this line the Bloch Wall, which is a neutral zone. This discovery, made by Dr. Davis and Walter Rawls, was later confirmed by the National Aeronautics and Space Administration.

We tend to forget that science, and particularly physics, is always evolving. There are always new discoveries, and theories are sometimes put aside for various reasons, whether financial or due to conflict between scientists. Scientists are people, after all, who want their particular theory to be right, and disagreements have taken place throughout the history of science.

For example, in the middle of the nineteenth century, Michael Faraday rejected the theory of effect at a distance as an explanation of magnetic action. He was the first to introduce the idea of lines of force, which is still an accepted theory. In 1851 he wrote: "I must express again my conviction that this concept is well founded.

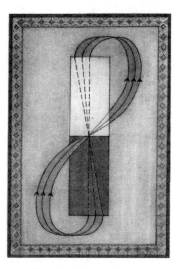

Fig. 16. Figure Eight Distribution

41

There is a clear advantage to using the idea of lines of force to explain magnetic action. All aspects of magnetic action observed in our experiments, that is, all concrete aspects, are easily explained and represented by lines of force." Another well-known English scientist of the same period, Sir George Airy, wrote the following four years later: "I must say that I find it altogether impossible to imagine that anyone who knows that numerical results confirm this theory [action at a distance] would hesitate an instant in choosing between the clear and simple action it outlines and the vague notion of lines of force."

Whichever theory of magnetism distribution you choose to accept, remember that induction lines enter at one pole and come out the other. As we said at the beginning of the book, we designate "north" the pole where lines of force enter and "south" the pole where they exit. Therefore, the south pole is associated with a positive charge and the north pole with a negative charge.

As for what happens inside a magnet, even the experts do not really know. It is difficult to observe the path of force lines inside a magnet. Some believe the lines form a bundle that follows a straight path parallel to the magnetic field. Others, like Davis, think the path is a vortex, with a 180° inversion at the center of the magnet. In any case, the external magnetic field is what interests us in this book. We will leave the rest to the experts.

DIFFERENCES BETWEEN NORTH AND SOUTH POLES

Experience shows that there are important differences between the north and south poles of magnets—aside from the fact that induction lines enter at one pole and exit at the other—especially in terms of their effects on living beings. We will discuss those effects in chapter 4. But everyone agrees that north and south magnetic forces are complementary. In physics terms, they are said to be opposed and "indissociable."

Many phenomena resemble magnetism in their characteristics.

We have only to think of electricity. A positive electric charge can be compared to the force of a magnet's south pole and a negative electric charge to its north pole. In the field of magnetism there are induction lines, whereas in the field of electricity there are lines of force. Similarly, heat can be associated with the south pole and cold with the north pole. Different people make different associations between magnets and various other phenomena. Some associate magnetism with traditional Chinese or Indian (Ayurvedic) medicine, Vedic astrology *(jyotish)*, or Vedic palmistry *(samudrik shastra)*. All of these associations are facets of the same reality, presented from different perspectives. Table 3 shows the most common associations with the different sections of a magnet.

TABLE 3: CHARACTERISTICS AND TERMS ASSOCIATED WITH THE POLES

NORTH	NEUTRAL AREA	SOUTH
Properties		
Negative	Neutral	Positive
Female	Hermaphrodite	Male
Cold	Warm	Hot
Counterclockwise		Clockwise
Centripetal		Centrifugal
Alkaline		Acid
Passive		Active
Effects		
Restrains, slows		Accelerates
Calms, reduces activity		Excites, activates
Attracts		Repels
Correspondence		
Electron	Neutron	Proton
Yin	*Rajas*	Yang
Sattwa	Air, ether	*Tamas*
Earth, water	Mercury, Saturn	Fire
Venus, moon, Jupiter		Mars, sun

MAGNETS AVAILABLE ON THE MARKET

Magnets and magnetized products can be purchased at hardware stores or pharmacies, through a manufacturer, or from scientific- or school-supply retailers. Objects magnetized for therapeutic purposes can include anything from knee guards to insoles, bracelets, belts, and mattresses. However, the strength and polarity of these products are not usually indicated. Therefore, one should try to obtain such information beforehand to avoid buying ineffective or inappropriate products.

Magnets sold separately come in various sizes and shapes, are made of various materials, and have different strengths.

MAGNETS OF DIFFERENT STRENGTHS

When a magnet is purchased from a school-supply catalog, the strength of the magnetic field is rarely indicated. Sometimes the catalog indicates "strong" or "very strong" but nothing more precise. The strength of magnets sold in hardware stores is given in pounds rather than gauss. For instance, a magnet 5 cm in diameter can have 25 lb strength, which means it can lift a 25 lb weight, such as a bag of nails. It is possible to measure the force of a magnet's field with a magnetometer, but these instruments are rather expensive and hard to find. Table 4 shows the equivalencies established by Dr. Davis between magnet strengths expressed in gauss and in pounds.

TABLE 4

Pounds	Gauss
2	500–600
5	900–1,200
15	1,500
25	2,000
50	3,500–4,500

Source: A. R. Davis, *Anatomy of Biomagnetics*, p. 38

MAGNETS OF VARIOUS SHAPES

Magnets come in several different shapes, and each shape is suited to different uses. The flat round models with a hole, available in hardware stores, are used mainly to lift weights. Their strength varies and is usually given in pounds. There are also flat rectangular magnets, with or without a hole; cylindrical magnets; and horseshoe magnets. Some are very flat and pliable, like those used to attach notes to refrigerator doors. Some are even sold on 2 cm wide tape, with both polarities on the same side. There are also tiny star-shaped magnets, slightly curved ones, and many other shapes and sizes.

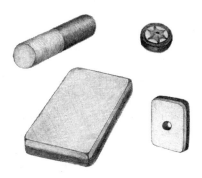

Fig. 17. Magnets of Different Shapes

HOW TO IDENTIFY THE POLES OF A MAGNET

It is not difficult to obtain magnets. However, the poles of most available magnets are rarely identified or are identified in different ways. So how can we tell which is north and which is south?

It's really very simple. One could use a magnetometer, which would also indicate strength in gauss, but, as we said, that instrument is expensive and difficult to find. So we recommend two simple and inexpensive methods. Because the first method involves the use of a compass, we will preface our description of that method with some useful information about compasses.

DISCOVERY OF THE COMPASS

The Chinese were the first to observe that a mineral tied to a piece of wood floating on water always turns in the same direction. This observation led to the invention of the compass, which consists of a magnetic needle mounted on a metal stem that is able to rotate freely around its support. The earth's magnetism is the force that acts on the needle. Ancient documents show that the compass was used by Chinese sailors as early as 1100, by Arab merchants around 1220, and by Vikings in 1250.

Early versions of the compass were improved by placing the needle and stem in an air-filled box, and improvements continued to be made over time. For instance, scientists discovered that the vibrations of the magnetic needle produced electric current, and that this current could be used to reduce vibration, which resulted in the invention of the shock-absorbent induction compass. The use of a liquid is now the most effective method of reducing magnetic needle vibrations in compasses. One can purchase excellent, inexpensive compasses at most sports equipment stores. (It is important to remember that in orienteering, magnetic and geographic poles do not coincide.)

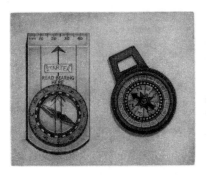

Fig. 18. Compasses

FINDING THE POLES OF A MAGNET WITH A COMPASS

As indicated, the first method for identifying the poles of a magnet involves the use of a compass. Because electric fields produce a magnetic field, it is important when using this method to keep at least 60 cm away from any electric equipment so you can identify the poles as accurately as possible.

First, turn the compass so that the magnetic needle points to the word "north" written on the edge of the compass. Bring one side of your magnet directly up to the compass needle. If the needle does not move, it means that the side of the magnet facing the compass is the north magnetic pole, since the compass needle points north. Place an "N" or some other mark on the north end of the magnet with indelible ink or nail polish. (Regardless of the method you choose, make sure you remember it.) However, if the compass needle spins halfway around (180°), it means that the side of the magnet facing the compass is the south magnetic pole.

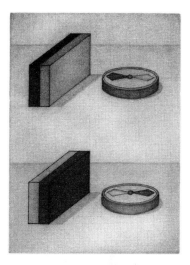

FINDING THE POLES WITHOUT A COMPASS

The second method of identifying the poles involves hanging a magnet so it can spin freely.

Fig. 19. Identifying the Poles of a Magnet Using a Compass

Please note that although it is easy to hang a perforated magnet by a thin but solid thread, with solid magnets the thread must be tied carefully around the middle of the magnet, in a state of balance; otherwise, the results may not be accurate.

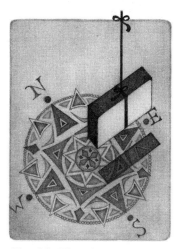

Fig. 20. Identifying the Poles of a Magnet Without Using a Compass

When you hang the magnet from a door frame, it will spin, turning first in one direction and then another; then, in a few minutes it will gradually slow down and stop completely. Do not interfere with the movement of the magnet until it comes to rest. If you know where north and south are in the room, even approximately, you will observe that the end of the magnet that ends up facing north geographically is the magnetic south pole (since that pole is attracted by the north).

Again, place the letter "N" or some other mark on the north end of the magnet with something indelible. Remember to use the same code to mark all your magnets, for example, the letter "N" or a specific color for the north pole.

Both of these methods for identifying magnetic poles are equally accurate and will produce the same results.

MAINTENANCE OF PERMANENT MAGNETS

Permanent magnets are rather delicate and easily broken. They should be handled with care and never dropped or knocked against other objects or hard surfaces because they can become chipped or lose energy if they are handled roughly.

Permanent magnets are also adversely affected by intense heat. They gradually lose their strength when heated, but only temporarily. However, above a certain temperature (350°C), most magnets lose their magnetic power completely and permanently. This critical temperature, the Curie point, varies depending on the metal. Therefore, magnets should not be left in a car in the summer, or in the hot sun. It is also wise to protect them from the cold, although they seem to tolerate cold better than heat.

Permanent magnets can lose strength over time. To avoid this, when storing magnets the two poles should be connected with a keeper, or small piece of metal (e.g., a sheet of tin, steel, or iron). This creates a closed circuit and maintains the original magnetic strength of the magnet.

WARNINGS ABOUT MAGNETS

Magnets should not be left near audio or video cassettes, because they can cause the cassettes to be erased. They can have the same effect on magnetized cards (bank cards, credit cards, bus passes, etc.), and they should not be used near people wearing pacemakers or defibrillators, because they can disturb the functioning of these devices.

Chapter Four

BIOMAGNETISM

Biomagnetism is the science that studies the effects of magnets on living organisms, that is, plants, animals, and human beings.

Before the beginning of this century, practitioners of magnet therapy applied either pole of the magnet interchangeably, or they applied both poles, as in the case of U-shaped magnets. At that time, it was not known that polarity makes a significant difference in the effect of the magnet. The specific effects of the south pole on living beings (and consequently the effects of the north pole) were discovered accidentally by Dr. Davis in 1936 in a small Florida laboratory. By chance, a small cardboard box containing compost and some fishing-bait earthworms were left near a strong horseshoe magnet. Two similar boxes were lying a little farther away, outside the field of the magnet.

After twenty-four hours, it was noticed that the worms in the first box had eaten through the cardboard and gathered close to the south pole of the magnet, whereas the other worms had not left their boxes. The experiment was subsequently repeated under the same conditions and produced the same results. (The experiment would take longer today because cardboard is now coated to delay deterioration.) In subsequent experiments, the temperature of the room was altered, different strengths of magnets were used, different magnetic poles were tried, a control group was introduced, and food and water were placed in the boxes. After twelve days, the following results were observed: Worms exposed to the south pole were longer, fatter, and more active, and they had also reproduced. In contrast, those exposed to the north pole were quite inactive and thin, and several had died. The results of the control group did not change.

IMPORTANT FACTORS IN BIOMAGNETISM

As you can see, in the study of biomagnetism the difference between the effects of the two poles is an important consideration. Other significant factors include the strength of the magnetic field, the length of exposure, the size of the surface area exposed, and the source of the magnetic field. We will discuss each of these factors separately.

THE MAGNETIC POLES

Remember that magnetic lines of force go in at the north pole and come out at the south pole. As a result, the two poles have different effects: The north pole soothes and the south pole energizes. These different effects must be kept in mind when doing experiments with magnets or when using them for particular purposes.

STRENGTH OF THE MAGNETIC FIELD

The law of pharmacological effect (the Arndt-Schulz law) also applies to magnetism: A low-intensity stimulus strengthens vital activity, a medium to strong stimulus tends to obstruct that activity, and a very strong stimulus stops or destroys it. Thus, the strength of the magnetic field is another important consideration. Magnetic field strength can be classified as follows: weak, less than 10 gauss; medium, 10 to 500 gauss; strong, 500 to 2,000 gauss; or very strong, over 2,000 gauss.

LENGTH OF EXPOSURE

The length of exposure, in combination with the strength of the magnetic field, is another contributing factor. For example, a strong magnet can be used for a very brief period (from a few seconds to a few minutes), or a weaker magnet can be used for a longer period (several hours or more), with different effects. The length of exposure can be brief (a few minutes to a few hours), medium (a few days), or long (several months or even years).

SIZE OF THE SURFACE AREA EXPOSED

Sometimes one magnet or several small magnets are applied directly on a specific area, such as a finger or a knee. In such cases, the treatment is local and the magnetism acts on the limited area only. At other times a larger area might be covered, through the use of bigger magnets or several smaller magnets. This type of treatment is called general because it acts on the whole body rather than a specific area. Therefore, the type of treatment used is often directly related to the surface area to be exposed to magnetism. In biomagnetism, "local treatment" refers to the application of magnetism to a restricted surface and "general treatment" refers to the application of magnetism to a large surface.

SOURCE OF THE MAGNETIC FIELD

The magnetic fields produced by permanent magnets can have very different effects from those produced by electromagnets. Therefore, the source of the magnetic field must also be taken into account. The main difference between the effect of permanent magnets and the effect of electromagnets can be summarized as follows:

Permanent magnets are characterized by a fixed magnetic field, so the intensity of magnetic current cannot be regulated; also, the poles of permanent magnets can be separated in certain situations. Electromagnets are characterized by a variable magnetic field, so the intensity of an electromagnet's magnetic current can be regulated; their poles cannot be separated; and they produce electric field effects in addition to magnetic field effects. (Please note that despite this discussion of the differences between permanent magnets and electromagnets, hereafter we will discuss the therapeutic application of permanent magnets only.)

As we have seen, in biomagnetism several factors have to be taken into consideration. It is because of the many variables involved that experiments in biomagnetism are sometimes seen as unscientific, for their authors can sometimes leave out important details. For instance, it is not enough to report that a 600-gauss magnet relieves pain; where it has been placed, for how long, how often, and at which pole are all important factors.

TABLE 5: MAGNET USE—MAIN POINTS TO REMEMBER

Pole	Unipolar: north and south
	Bipolar: both poles together
Surface area exposed	Local treatment
	General treatment
Length of exposure	Brief: a few minutes or hours
	Medium: a few days
	Long: a few months or years
Strength of magnetic field	Weak: less than 10 gauss
	Medium: 10 to 500 gauss
	Strong: 500 to 2,000 gauss
	Very strong: over 2,000 gauss

EFFECTS OF MAGNETISM ON CELLS

Magnetism has an effect on all living organisms, regardless of size. Because living organisms are often classified according to the kingdom they belong to (unicellular, vegetable, or animal), we will use the same classifications in this book. Although human beings do not constitute a separate category according to the strict definition of "kingdom," we will refer to them as a fourth subdivision.

Several studies have been done on the effects of magnetism at the cellular level, both with fixed magnetic fields (permanent magnets) and variable fields (electromagnets). Experiments on primitive organisms demonstrate that several of these organisms have remarkable sensitivity to the earth's magnetic field, due to very efficient receptors. The existence of bacteria sensitive to magnetism was discovered in 1975 by Richard P. Blakemore, who was then a student at the University of Massachusetts at Amherst. Since then many different types of such bacteria have been identified. Subsequent studies have confirmed the presence of magnetically charged magnetite grains in these bacteria. For instance, some bacteria living in riverbed silt normally swim downward; but if they're exposed to a magnetic field opposed to that of the earth, they start to swim upward. Moreover, bacteria living in the southern hemisphere (where the direction of the vertical axis of the magnetic field is opposite to that in the northern hemisphere) start to swim upward when they are taken north to the United States. In contrast, in Brazil, where the magnetic field is horizontal, silt bacteria swim in all directions.

Other experiments have demonstrated the effects of magnetism on macromolecules, rods in the retina, muscle fibers, and photosynthetic systems. Magnetic fields also exert effects on water, a subject we will deal with in chapter 6.

EFFECTS OF MAGNETISM ON PLANTS

In Florida, numerous experiments have been conducted on the effects of magnetic fields on seeds both before and after germination. Those experiments show that seeds planted in the earth with their tips pointing south sprout more quickly and produce plants that are more vigorous. The use of magnets has also been shown to increase fertility, rejuvenate tissues, and promote resistance to disease. However, experiments have also shown that a weak magnetic field is sufficient and that prolonged exposure can actually produce the opposite result.

Laboratory analyses reveal the many significant effects the south pole of a magnet can have on living organisms: Exposure to the south pole has been shown to raise temperature, stimulate oxygen release, and facilitate the absorption of carbon dioxide, organic elements, and fertilizers. Plants have longer and more numerous roots, and they grow faster. Germination is rapid, followed by improved development of the roots and a sudden and remarkable emergence of the external portion of the plant. Beets produce more sugar, as do yams, and peanuts produce more oil. The amino acid content of proteins is higher than in nonmagnetized plants, even if the latter have been fertilized. Two American horticulturists, Dr. A. A. Boe and Dr. D. K. Salunke, have noted that when green tomatoes are exposed to the south pole of a magnet, they ripen four to six times faster.

The north pole has been shown to have the opposite effect on seeds; plants exposed to this pole are stunted and less fertile than normal. However, experiments show that the north pole can cause tomatoes to produce less acid, which in some cases is advantageous. Try this experiment with three oranges (or lemons or grapefruit): Over a period of thirty-six hours, expose one of the oranges to the north pole of a magnet and another to the south pole, and keep the third away from the magnet as a control. At the end of the experiment, the fruit exposed to the north pole will taste the sweetest.

The following seed experiment was conducted by Dr. Davis's team.*

SEED EXPERIMENT

Length of exposure: 8, 10, 80, 100, and 280 hours.

Strength of field: not specified.

Unipolar: north or south pole.

Protocol: The seeds were placed in sealed envelopes glued to one end of a magnet (north or south) and clearly identified. A control group was kept in another room, far from any source of magnetism. Other factors such as

---

*Source: Albert Roy Davis and Walter C. Rawls, *Magnetism and Its Effects on the Living System* (Hicksville, N.Y.: Exposition Press, 1974), 29.

environment, temperature, pressure, and so on were kept uniform to allow for the experiment to be repeated.

Observations: Seeds exposed to the south pole of a magnet produced more vigorous plants than normal. Plants emerging from seeds exposed to the north pole were weak compared to the control group. Length of exposure was extremely important and dependent on the type of seed involved. For example, root vegetables such as radishes reacted better and faster to exposure to the south pole than other vegetables.

EFFECTS OF MAGNETISM ON ANIMALS

One summer day in 1995, I watched the surprising behavior of an insect that had landed on my arm. Since it was not in a hurry to fly away, I had time to observe it. It advanced on my arm, always in the same direction. I turned my arm to try to confuse it, but after a second or two it always found its way back and continued in the same direction, as if it had a compass in its brain. I played the game for a few minutes and then placed the insect on the grass.

The effect of magnetism on the directional sense of certain fish (e.g., sharks and rays) as well as on the movements of mollusks, the migration of birds, and the flight of bees has been observed for a long time. In the case of homing pigeons, this characteristic has been and is still used in the service of humanity. These pigeons will become disoriented when small magnets are attached to their heads. As with silt bacteria, particles of magnetically charged magnetite have been detected in all of these living creatures. And we now know that the brains of whales also contain magnetic particles, which help these animals to navigate.

After conducting experiments on plant seeds, Dr. Davis studied the possible effect of magnetism on prenatal development in small animals. The following experiment on eggs was conducted by Dr. Davis's team in a laboratory setting.*

---

*Source: Davis and Rawls, *Magnetism and Its Effects on the Living System*, pp. 33-35.

EGG EXPERIMENT

Length of exposure: not specified.

Strength of field: straight cylindrical magnets, 2,500 gauss.

Unipolar: north or south pole.

Protocol: Twenty-four fertilized chicken eggs, divided into three groups of eight; Group N exposed to the north pole, Group S exposed to the south pole, and control Group C not exposed. A separate magnet was used for each exposed egg. The exposed eggs were turned every three hours. Temperature was kept constant at 80°F for the duration of the experiment. After hatching, the chicks were placed in three separate cages. In each cage, there was a horseshoe magnet, 13 x 15 cm, with the poles 6.5 cm apart, as well as a fake magnet of the same size and shape.

Observations: The incubation period of the eggs exposed to the south pole was two to three days shorter than the incubation period of the control group; it was one to two days longer for eggs exposed to the north pole. After hatching, the chicks exposed to the south pole placed themselves, while still wet, between the poles of the horseshoe magnet and stayed there for about two minutes. After that, they moved as far from the magnet as possible. None of the chicks were fooled by the fake magnet. The chicks exposed to the north pole acted the same way, but stayed about three minutes longer in the magnetic field. The chicks that had not been exposed to any magnetic field waited until they were dry before entering the magnetic field and then stayed there between two and a half and three and a half minutes.

Similar experiments produced similar results. When eggs were exposed to the magnetism of the south pole for periods between thirty minutes and five hours, they hatched more quickly. If the exposure time was longer, not only was there no change in the time it took for the eggs to hatch, but the chicks were smaller at birth. Another experiment showed that chicks in a cage instinctively moved toward magnets but stayed there between five and seven minutes only. These chicks paid no attention to fake magnets placed in the cage.

Dr. Davis later studied the development of fowl (chickens and roosters) placed in a magnetic field. When the fowl were exposed to the south pole, they grew more quickly, became bigger, and reached their maturity stage faster; however, they seemed less intelligent. The fowl exposed to the north pole grew more slowly than those in the control group, were more aware of their environment, were leaner and more high strung, and ate less but drank more water. The fowl in the two groups showed remarkable differences in behavior. Once they reached maturity, the birds exposed to the south pole became aggressive even to the point of attacking and eating the other fowl in their group, becoming cannibalistic. In contrast, at maturity the birds exposed to the north pole drank less water but ate more without gaining weight, as if they had undergone a genetic change.

Several experiments were carried out on small mammals. One experiment on mice showed that when the females were exposed to the north pole of a magnet, they gave birth more easily and seemingly with less pain. Buryl Payne mentions that in another experiment mice were exposed to a 10,000-gauss magnet for thirty minutes a day for ten days and subsequently showed an increase of 4 to 11 percent in bone weight and 4 to 9 percent in bone length. The experiment was conducted with a control group, but the pole of the magnet used was not specified.

A Russian biologist succeeded in doubling the life span of flies by feeding them magnetized sugar. It has also been shown that the life span of a mouse can be prolonged by exposure to a magnetic field between 3,000 and 4,000 gauss, twice a day, for an hour each time.

Kathy Solis, an American scientist, conducted a four-year experiment in which she exposed animals to a 3,000-gauss bipolar magnetic field, and that experiment produced the following results: The number of erythrocytes (red blood cells) of the animals increased, and the number of leukocytes (white blood cells) decreased. Because red blood cells are the major carriers of oxygen in the body, an increase in their number stimulates vitality. But a decrease in the number of white blood cells is dangerous, because those cells are the foundation of the immune system. Before the experiment, the animals had been injected with cancer cells. The number of cancer cells seemed to decrease after the animals were exposed to the bipolar magnetic field, but the cancer reappeared when exposure to the bipolar magnetic field ceased.

Dr. Davis also conducted experiments in the field of cancer research, similar to those carried out by Kathy Solis, but he used a unipolar magnetic field instead. To work with unipolar (or separated) fields, the magnets used must be flat or long, and not of the horseshoe type, in which it is difficult to separate the poles. Dr. Davis usually used flat, 15 x 5 cm magnets, 1 cm thick. They are nonmetallic and retain their magnetizing power for about five years, after which they have to be recharged. These magnets are applied directly to the skin.

In Dr. Davis's experiments different types of cancer cells were injected into mice, rats, and other small animals. These animals were then exposed to 3,000-gauss unipolar magnetic fields. He observed that exposure to the north pole for forty-five to sixty minutes two or three times a day reduced infection and relieved pain, and that exposure to the south pole improved circulation, stimulated cell renewal in both healthy and cancerous cells, facilitated scarring when there was no infection, and improved digestion—in short, stimulated vital functions in general.

A study conducted by Rosemonde Mandeville, a doctor and researcher at the Armand Frappier Institute of Laval, Quebec, Canada, seems to indicate that magnetic fields are not a source of cancer, at least in rats. A type of rat particularly susceptible to cancer, type F-344, was used in the experiment. For two years, six groups of fifty rats were exposed for twenty hours a day to 60 Hz magnetic fields with intensities between 2 and 2,000 microtesla (0.02 to 20 gauss). This intensity is twenty thousand times higher than intensities produced by domestic appliances. The experiment was conducted as a double-blind study, meaning that the laboratory technician did not know the intensity of the fields and therefore could not bias the results. After the exposure, the tissue and organ cells of the three hundred rats were analyzed, and the results revealed that there was no significant statistical difference in the incidences of tumor between the groups of rats. However, although this study is reassuring, it does not totally eliminate the possibility that magnetic fields could stimulate the progress of already existing cancers, and therefore we cannot apply its results to humans.

Experimental data on fixed magnetic fields of intensities below 2 tesla (20,000 gauss) indicate the absence of irreversible effects on most growth factors, physiology, and behavior in higher species. Remember that 20,000-gauss magnets are very strong—much more powerful than magnets designed for domestic use.

EFFECTS OF MAGNETISM ON HUMAN BEINGS

Until recently, it was believed that humans did not have magnetic receptors like those found in primitive organisms and certain animals. However, a few years ago researchers at the California Institute of Technology, using very sensitive magnetometers, discovered magnetic particles in the human brain very similar to those found in several types of animals. These particles are tiny—one-millionth of a centimeter in diameter—which explains why they were not found earlier. They are scattered throughout the brain, particularly in the meninges, the membranes covering the brain. The total weight of the particles contained in the brain is about one-millionth of an ounce. As we said in chapter 3, certain parts of the human body, like the blood and the muscles, are paramagnetic; that is, they react weakly to magnetic fields. Therefore, it should not be surprising to discover that magnetic fields can affect human metabolism.

MAGNETIC FIELD DEFICIENCY SYNDROME

It is obvious that magnetic fields affect vital energy in humans, as they do in other mammals. It is interesting to note that the strength of the earth's magnetic field, the major source of magnetism to which we are exposed, has apparently diminished by half in the past five hundred years and now measures about 0.5 gauss. The strength of the field continues to decrease by about 5 percent every one hundred years and will probably disappear almost completely within two thousand years. In addition, the lifestyle of many North Americans and Europeans only serves to further weaken the effect of the magnetic field on humans: The skyscrapers and high-rise buildings in which we live and work and the cars in which we spend more and more time cut us off, at least partially, from the little earth magnetism that remains. The materials of modern buildings and cars, such as steel and iron, are ferromagnetic and, as such, intercept the magnetism emanating from the earth and deprive us of its effects.

It has been theorized that this shortage of magnetism could be the cause of various symptoms that afflict more and more people today. Dr. Kyoichi Nakagawa calls this deficiency Magnetic Field Deficiency Syndrome (MFDS). A syndrome is a set of symptoms or signs associated with a given pathological state that, by appearing together, indicate a possible diagnosis. Diagnosing syndromes can be difficult because the symptoms are often similar to those of other illnesses. In the case of MFDS, the symptoms can be mistaken for those of hypertension, diabetes, or ataxia, and the presence of MFDS can only be clearly established by its positive reaction to magnetic treatment.

In an article published in the *Japan Medical Journal* (no. 2745, December 4, 1976), Nakagawa presented the results of research he conducted over twenty years on the effects of magnetism on human beings. The various symptoms of MFDS he identified include stiffness of shoulders, back, and neck; diffuse lumbago; unexplained chest pain; frequent headaches and "heaviness" in the head; dizziness; unexplained insomnia; constant constipation; central nervous system imbalance, or ataxia; and general fatigue.

These symptoms can characterize conditions other than MFDS; they are often associated with hypertension, diabetes, or digestive problems. Therefore, MFDS can only be established if symptoms persist after the suspected traditional disease has been treated. In other words, the syndrome itself does not produce an objective pathology detectable by a routine medical exam. However, the subjective symptoms of MFDS, such as pain or stiffness, which are not measurable, will persist and fail to respond to any treatment other than one directly related to magnetic energy. Thus, a patient has to respond to a magnetism-based treatment for MFDS to be diagnosed with certainty.

As early as 1958, Dr. Nakagawa and his team published the results of tests conducted to observe the effect of magnetism on shoulder stiffness. He achieved great success with patients made to wear magnetic bracelets, and details concerning these tests were presented the following year at a conference on magnetism.

MAGNETIC OVERLOAD

Given the possible effects of a shortage of magnetism, it is reasonable to ask if an excess of magnetism might also have adverse effects on health. According to the World Health Organization (WHO), the answer is no. In 1987, the WHO published a two-hundred-page book in Geneva, Switzerland, entitled *Magnetic Fields: Environmental Health Criteria,* which recommends subsequent studies on the subject. The publication also refers to several research studies examining the biological effects of static and variable magnetic fields, including effects on molecular and cellular structure, tissues and organs, circulation, the nervous system, vision, physiological regulatory function, genes, reproduction, and growth. It also evaluates the health risk of magnetism and makes recommendations. According to the WHO, most biological functions are not significantly affected by static magnetic fields of less than 20,000 gauss (which is extremely high). However, in the studies they refer to, no distinction is made between the north and south poles.

Health and Welfare Canada has published a report on megametric electric and magnetic fields, which means fields of very high intensity. Given the advent of new technologies using very powerful magnets, such as cyclotrons, fusion reactors, magnetic levitation systems used in the transport industry and scrap metal yards, and more recently magnetic resonance machines used as medical diagnostic tools, it would be useful to establish standards limiting our exposure to very strong magnetic fields. However, for the moment, it seems no further research is being conducted on the effects of megametric magnetic fields on human beings.

Many of the experiments in the WHO publication involving biological organisms exposed to magnetic fields were done in vitro. However, effects on human health cannot be based solely on in vitro studies, because the effects seen in vitro will not necessarily appear in vivo. In vitro studies can make it possible to evaluate the toxicity of a certain substance and to define preventive measures to be included in safety norms, for example. However, it is not always possible to extrapolate from in vitro results to draw conclusions about human beings. Ideally, the health risks should be evaluated according to well-designed, well-conducted, and correctly analyzed studies. But, unfortunately, epidemiological studies on human beings exposed to magnetic fields often have the following drawbacks: The sample size is too small (not enough subjects), there is no control group, and there is a lack of information on external variables that could affect the study (exposure to other physical or chemical factors).

A number of other studies on this subject have been conducted all over the world—in Germany, Canada, the United States, Finland, Italy, Japan, and several other countries. Researchers have examined the effects of magnetism on cells, glands, nerves, and liquids. Some studies have examined magnetic effects on biochemical activity, mutagenesis (the process that introduces a mutation), blood chemistry, and hypertension. In the case of superior-scale organisms exposed to static magnetic fields, the two types of effects observed can be explained by plausible mechanisms of interaction: induction of electric potential and of magnetohydrodynamic effects in the circulation system and direct stimulation of nerve and muscle cells. We will examine these two types of effects next.

THE CIRCULATORY SYSTEM

Magnetism acts on paramagnetic elements in the body, especially the blood, and it is mainly through the circulatory system that the effects of magnetism are dispersed throughout the body. Therefore, it is important to understand how the human circulation system functions.

The human body contains 5 to 6 liters (10 to 12 pints) of blood, which are pumped to every organ of the body. Arteries, arterioles, and capillaries carry oxygen and other essential elements to those organs. The same capillaries then take back the used blood, which carries toxins and waste products, and empty it into the veins. On its way back to the heart, the blood goes through the kidneys, where it is filtered, then through the lungs, where it is recharged with oxygen. The blood, now refilled with fresh oxygen, reaches the heart, from which it is sent off again to the organs.

Human blood is composed of blood cells (45 percent) and plasma cells (55 percent). Blood cells contain mainly red cells (erythrocytes), white cells (leukocytes), and platelets. A red cell functions like a small container for a substance called hemoglobin, which gives blood its particular color. A hemoglobin molecule contains enough iron (4 atoms/10,000) to make red cells slightly paramagnetic and therefore subject to the effects of magnetic fields. Moreover, red blood cells are the major oxygen transporters in the body. When the body's red cell count is considerably diminished, or when the hemoglobin content of those cells, and consequently their iron content, is too low, the body does not receive enough oxygen to maintain an adequate level of energy. Anemia is a condition where there is loss of energy due to lack of iron. It has been shown that magnets can increase blood conductivity slightly, and ionized blood can improve blood circulation and stabilize high or low blood pressure. Therefore, magnetized blood can carry more oxygen to the cells; in other words, it can make more energy available to tissues and organs, which perform better as a result.

Sometimes arteries become partially obstructed by fat deposits or accumulations of calcium or cholesterol. Because blood flow is impeded, oxygen supply, as well as the supply of other essential nutrients, is diminished. Fortunately, it has been observed that magnetism activates and accelerates blood circulation. Magnetized hemoglobin not only facilitates better oxygen supply, but also allows better waste elimination. Internal organs that are well supplied with what they need tire less quickly. In England, the teams working in the Delawarr Laboratories with an electromagnetic field produced by a solenoid have observed the following in the blood of human subjects: a reduction of cholesterol levels, a lower white blood cell count, an increase in the secretion of cortical hormones, faster coagulation, and a decrease in blood pressure (from 140/90 mm Hg before treatment to 125/80 mm Hg after three weeks of treatment).*

Improved blood circulation is always beneficial because a better oxygen supply contributes to optimal functioning of all organs in the body and strengthens the immune system. Magnetism also reduces cholesterol levels and calcium deposits in blood vessels. Magnets do not cure, but they do have a synergetic effect: They allow the body to regain balance and better defend itself against external invasion.

THE NERVOUS SYSTEM

Magnetism also has remarkable effects on the nervous system. Dr. Davis in his *Anatomy of Biomagnetics,*** and Dr. A. K. Bhattacharya in *Power in a Magnet to Heal,*[†] have long claimed that north pole energy has an anesthetic effect on pain, and we now know how magnetism exerts this effect on the nervous system.

---

*The appendix of *Biomagnetism* by G. W. de la Warr (Oxford, UK: Delawarr Laboratories, 1967), presents detailed hematological findings (red and white cell count, sedimentation, granulocytes, monocytes, etc.) obtained during preliminary studies on the effects of magnetic fields on human tissues and organs.

**Albert Roy Davis, *Anatomy of Biomagnetics* (San Lorenzo, Puerto Rico: Litolibros, 1974).

†Dr. A. K. Bhattacharya and Ralph U. Sierra, *Power in a Magnet to Heal* (Naihati, India, 1976), Third Edition 1985.

The basic building block of the nervous system is the nerve cell, or neuron. These cells produce a form of energy that passes through their membranes. Ions are carried outside the body by axons, which are a kind of prolongation of the neurons. Axons are usually covered with a coating called myelin, which insulates them and increases the conduction speed of nervous influx (the name given to this positive ion discharge). Neurons carry impulses between the body periphery and the central nervous system. This

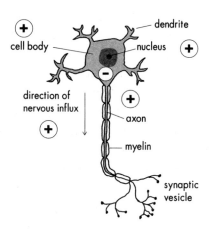

Fig. 21. Nerve Cell
(internal charge is negative)

system is very complex. Some neurons are linked by connections called synapses, and it is believed that in the brain and spinal cord there are over ten trillion such synapses. So imagine how complex neuron activity must be in the brain and spinal cord!

Sensory neurons react to touch, pressure, pain, temperature, position, muscular tension, chemical concentration, light, and other mechanical stimuli. They make us aware of our internal and external environment and of changes taking place within them. When nerve cells are stimulated, they send messages to the brain. An electrochemical impulse travels along the nerve, and its passage is facilitated or inhibited by the presence or absence of synapses. When the brain finally receives the impulse, it interprets the message and responds to it. The response is either voluntary or involuntary (reflex).

Unlike blood cells, nerve cells have a negative internal charge and a positive external charge. When nerve endings are stimulated, the external positive charge becomes very powerful. Under this pressure, the cell membrane opens for a fraction of a second, letting positive ions pass into the interior of the cell (charges always travel from the positive to the negative). The positive charge inside the cell tends to transmit itself to the adjacent nerve cell, and so on. The charge travels all along the nerve path to the brain. This nervous influx is a kind of signal. To feel pain, there must be stimulation of nerve endings, and the brain must be informed of this stimulation and interpret it. If the nerve is cut, if something else stops the influx from reaching the brain, or if the influx is too weak, no pain will be felt.

This explains the anesthetic effect of the north pole. When the north pole of a magnet is applied to the skin next to nerve endings, the negative energy of the magnet and the positive energy of the nerve cells attract each other. A bioelectric exchange takes place, from the positive toward the negative. In other words, the positive charge at the surface of the nerve cells is reduced because part of it is carried away toward the negative pole of the magnet, so that less energy travels to the brain. Therefore, the brain receives a less intense message and signals a reduction of pain; an anesthetic effect has taken place. Menstrual cramps are a good example of a problem that responds well to the application of the north pole of a magnet. The same is true of muscle and joint pain having no specific cause or, in some cases, caused by excessive physical exertion.

THE ENDOCRINE SYSTEM

The endocrine system also responds to magnetism. Whereas the nervous system acts directly on muscles and glands (which govern rapid somatic activity), the endocrine system exerts a slower effect. It acts on cells by means of chemical substances called hormones, which are secreted directly into the blood. These hormones produce a specific effect on certain types of cells. Each cell has receptors that recognize only the molecules of hormones intended specifically for it and that draw the hormone molecules out of the blood circulatory system. Some endocrine glands are activated by the nervous system and others by chemical changes in the body.

Hormones and neurotransmitters are compared as follows:

Hormones of the endocrine system and neurotransmitters
in the nervous system have a similar function: they carry

messages between the cells of the body. A neurotransmitter carries messages between neurons that are next to each other, so its effect is localized. A hormone, on the other hand, can travel over long distances in the body and produce various effects on several types of cells. Despite this difference, these chemical messengers have something in common, because some of them perform both types of functions. For example, adrenaline and norepinephrine act as neurotransmitters when they are released by neurons, and as hormones when they are produced by suprarenal glands.*

Hormonal secretions can be regulated and even improved by the effects of magnetism because the capillaries surrounding the glands are part of the blood circulatory system, which has been shown to be affected by magnetism. Dilating the capillaries allows better transmission of hormones to all parts of the body and therefore improves overall health. Because glands sometimes stimulate hormone secretion in other glands, the effect produced by regulating hormonal function can be astonishing. Dr. H. L. Bansal claims that reduced functioning of the pituitary gland (which is responsible for dwarfism) can be corrected by applying magnetic fields combined with other methods of treatment, such as homeopathy, if the condition is detected early enough (before age fourteen or fifteen).

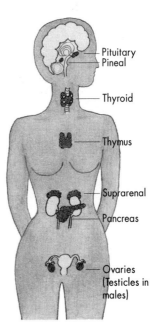

Fig. 22. Endocrine System

---

*Translation of a quote from R. L. Atkinson, R. C. Atkinson, E. E. Smith, and D. J. Bem, eds., *Introduction à la psychologie,* 3rd edition (Montreal: Les Éditions de la Chenelière, 1994), 59.

OTHER CURATIVE EFFECTS OF MAGNETS

SCARRING

Magnetism acts not only on the blood, nerves, and glands, but also on the cells. In one of his patients, Holger Hanneman observed that collagen formation was symmetrical and at a right angle with the incision along the section treated with magnets, whereas along the nontreated section scarring occurred in a chaotic, haphazard pattern. He also discovered that magnetism can help to restore elasticity in scar tissue, particularly and often quite remarkably in burn cases. However, Hanneman cautions that because research shows that the south pole increases vital energy in all living beings, including microbes and bacteria, only the north pole should be used where there is infection.

CANCER

Some doctors have pointed to the beneficial effects of magnetism in cancer treatment. Dr. John Pole, professor of Pediatric Hematology-Oncology at the University of Florida, reports on a magnetic treatment of bone marrow that has tripled the survival rate of children suffering from neuroblastoma, a cancer of the nervous system that generally produces abdominal tumors and spreads to the bone marrow. The treatment consists of injecting magnetic particles into extracted bone marrow, where the particles adhere to cancer cells only. Then the fluid is "strained" using special magnetic equipment to separate healthy cells from cancer cells. The fluid is frozen and is reinjected after the patient has received chemotherapy or radiotherapy. The reinjected fluid is disease free, since it no longer contains cancer cells, and it is also compatible, thereby eliminating the risk of rejection.

According to Dr. Robert Seeger, professor of Pediatric Hematology-Oncology at the University of Southern California School of Medicine, a two-year-old child diagnosed with neuroblastoma was in perfect health three years after receiving magnetic-based treatment. Once again, it was observed that while the application of magnetic fields was not a cure, it significantly reinforced and enhanced the healing process. Nearly 50 percent of children with neuroblastoma, which is fatal in 90 percent of cases, lived an average of two years without recurrence of disease following magnetic treatment.

It has also been reported that breast cancer has been success-fully treated with Neomax magnets, which are 4,000-gauss magnets made of iron, boron, and neodymium. About the size of a quarter and weighing about 30 g, these magnets were designed in 1983 based on Professor Göesta Wollin's specifications and are manu-factured and marketed by the Sumitomo Special Metals Company of Japan. Professor Wollin used this new product successfully in the treatment of three breast cancer patients who wore Neomax magnets for four months on neck chains, but not directly on the tumor. Professor Wollin believes this method of using these supermagnets has a beneficial effect on the whole body. He clari-fies that "this type of treatment does not damage healthy cells because healthy cells have different electromagnetic potential than cancer cells."* He also points out that magnet therapy consti-tutes the first new type of cancer treatment since the advent of chemotherapy forty years ago.

OTHER EFFECTS

Other researchers have reported that fractures heal in signifi-cantly shorter periods when treated with permanent or electro-magnets. This could be due to the fact that the activity of calcium ions (as well as that of magnesium, sodium, and potassium ions) is altered by magnetic fields. And, of course, calcium is an essential element in bone formation.

Some claim that magnetism helps stabilize enzyme activity and keep the body's acid/base balance at an ideal level. Patients report that treatment is usually followed by a sensation of calm, and that treatment of the colon usually results in bowel movements, as well

---

*Göesta Wollin and Eric Enby, *Curing Cancer with Supermagnets,* summary of a fifty-seven page report presented by G. Wollin on November 20, 1987 at Chalmers University of Technology (Göteborg, Sweden).

as better elimination function in both the urinary tract and the digestive system, especially if magnetized water is also used. (Magnetized water will be examined in detail in chapter 6.)

We probably do not yet know all the specific effects that magnetic fields can have on human metabolism, but what we already know indicates that magnetism has definite beneficial effects on several vital functions. Although there are some instances in which magnetic fields are not recommended (which will be discussed in the next chapter), research shows that magnetic fields have practically no side effects and are therefore very useful in the treatment of physical ailments. Every home should be equipped with magnets and use them to maintain and improve the health of the family.

The following is a partial list of conditions that have been observed to respond to magnetic treatment:

Alzheimer's disease
Anxiety
Arthritis (certain types)
Asthma
Backache
Bladder weakness
Bruises
Bursitis
Cancer (certain types)
Cataracts
Cerebral palsy
Diabetes
Diverticulitis
Dizziness
Fractures
Gall bladder disorders
Glandular imbalance
Glaucoma
Headaches

Kidney diseases
Liver diseases
Menstrual cramps
Multiple sclerosis
Pancreatic disorders
Prostate disorders
Reflux
Schizophrenia
Sinus congestion
Spleen disorders

Given that the effects of the north and the south pole are different, magnets must be used carefully. Always bear in mind that the south pole enhances the growth and proliferation of cells, whether they are healthy or not, and that using the wrong pole could cause tumor growth or stimulate bacterial proliferation. Therefore, in case of doubt, the south pole should not be used at all.

Chapter Five

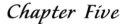

MAGNET THERAPY

Please read this chapter carefully before you begin to practice magnet therapy. It provides a practical perspective on magnetic treatments and contains essential information and guidance on the proper application of magnetic fields. The information provided in the "Warnings" section below is extremely important and should be reviewed on a regular basis. Always make sure the selected magnetic treatment is appropriate for the person and condition in question.

It is important to understand the limitations of magnet therapy, as well as its recognized benefits. Magnet therapy should not be used to treat serious conditions that require specialized medical treatment and could involve complications. We strongly recommend you always check with a doctor to see if the magnet therapy you are planning to use is compatible with other treatments you or the patient may be receiving. Magnet therapy will not solve all health problems or perform miracles, nor is it a substitute for a healthy and balanced lifestyle and good dietary habits. However, it has been shown that when used judiciously magnet therapy can greatly assist the body's constant striving to maintain balance. This being the case, we should take advantage of its benefits.

WARNINGS

It is important to take care of the magnets you use in magnet therapy: They should be handled carefully and protected from shocks, extreme temperatures, and demagnetization. However, it is also important to take care of the person being treated, and we recommend that you always observe the rules outlined below when using magnets:

Never use magnets on someone who has a pacemaker.

Do not apply strong magnets near the heart without proper medical advice.

Do not use magnets on pregnant women or on children under two years of age.

Do not apply strong magnets to the abdomen after a large meal, as doing so can alter gastric acidity and interfere with digestion. It is best to wait at least two hours after a meal before beginning magnetic treatment.

Never use only the south pole around the head, or where there is infection or tumor.

When you expose a person to the south pole of a magnet, finish the treatment with the polarity-balancing procedure described in the "Treatments" section of this chapter.

Be careful about the duration of treatment when using the north pole only, as prolonged use of the north pole of a strong magnet can cause fatigue in certain people.

Always monitor carefully the reactions of the person you are treating. Some people respond more quickly and strongly to magnetic treatment. If symptoms like yawning, a heavy head, tingling, or nausea occur, stop the treatment immediately.

NORTH POLE OR SOUTH POLE?
PROPERTIES OF THE TWO POLES

Table 3 lists the properties generally associated with each of the magnetic poles. These poles also have specific properties that affect human metabolism and therefore are used for specific purposes. Many years of empirical experiment and observation have proven the different and specific effects that each pole has on the human body.

You can easily conduct your own experiments and confirm these observations. For instance, if you apply the north pole of a

TABLE 6: THERAPEUTIC PROPERTIES OF THE TWO POLES

North Pole	South Pole
Sedative	Excites, increases activity
Soothes nervous pain	Soothes muscle pain by producing heat
Reduces inflammation	Stimulates infection
Stimulates healing process	Stimulates all life forms, including germs, viruses, and bacteria
Controls infection by slowing reproduction of microorganisms	Stimulates tumor growth
Stops tumor growth	Stimulates growth and maturation
Slows growth and maturation processes	Stimulates cellular activity in all biological organisms
Slows metabolism	
Impedes life by slowing cellular activity	Increases energy
Alkaline, reduces acidity	Increases acidity
Reduces calcium deposits in blood	Increases calcium deposits in blood
Stops bleeding	Increases bleeding
Attracts red and white blood cells essential for healing	Increases number of red blood cells
	Causes dilation of blood vessels
Causes constriction of blood vessels	Stimulates fluid circulation and congestion
Reduces liquid retention by stimulating elimination	Allows muscle relaxation
	Decreases blood pressure
Causes muscle contraction	Increases hydrogen ion concentration
Increases blood pressure	Stimulates cardiac activity, increases pulse
Regulates the quantity of oxygen in tissues, increases oxygen absorption	Stimulates tissue regeneration
Slows cardiac activity, slows pulse	
Reduces ulcers	
Improves concentration	

500-gauss magnet to a mosquito bite, slight skin irritation, or light burn, you will find that the pain disappears in just a few minutes, as if by magic. These simple experiments will convince you that the north pole of a magnet effectively soothes pain.

We have seen that magnets can affect blood circulation, the nervous system, the endocrine system, cell growth, digestion, elimination—in short, the entire metabolism. However, experts have observed that different effects are achieved when only the north pole or only the south pole is applied, or when both poles are used together. These observations are consistent and confirm the experimental results of other researchers. Table 6 summarizes the properties that researchers and practitioners most often associate with each pole. As you can see, the list is long, and no doubt other properties could be added.

Since each pole performs a different function, it is important to use the proper pole in unipolar treatment. Because of its activating properties, the south pole must be used with more caution than the north pole. When in doubt, it is better to avoid south pole treatment than to risk unwanted complications.

CHOOSING THE RIGHT TIME FOR TREATMENT

Another important factor in magnet therapy is the timing of treatments, which should be in harmony with the biological rhythms of the organs being treated. Whether you are using magnet therapy, acupuncture, or shiatsu, it is always preferable to treat an organ in the phase of its most intense activity.

The theory of energetic rhythms is not new. It is an integral aspect of Ayurvedic medicine, an ancient science that dates back to post-Vedic periods.* Traditional Chinese medicine refers to "the hour of the liver"—three o'clock in the morning—as a time when the depressed have trouble sleeping, a theory that has now been confirmed and explained by liver cell research and data. Periodic phenomena were also cited in ancient Greek writings: Hippocrates

---

*Ayurveda, or "the science of life," has its origins in the ancient sacred texts of India, either the Upanishad or a branch of the Atharva Veda.

and others noted that episodes of depression tended to increase in the spring and autumn months, and such seasonal depression is well documented by scientists today.

Chronobiology is a relatively recent branch of biological study that includes time periods and rhythms in its understanding and description of biological phenomena. Although it has been a recognized discipline only since the late 1950s, it is now enjoying rapid growth. Chronobiology demonstrates that rhythmic activity is a basic property of living matter, and that the functioning of each organ is subject to a daily twenty-four-hour biological cycle. The sleep/wakefulness cycle is a clear example of this circadian rhythm. Although scientists theorize that the mechanism responsible for controlling this biological rhythm could be located in the central nervous system, they have yet to discover its exact nature and location.

Some pharmacological research takes the human body's natural biological rhythms into account, for instance in studies measuring the toxic-effect variations of a given organ's sensitivity. "These studies show that the time when a medication is administered can be as important a factor as the dosage. Therefore, it becomes possible to determine the period when the medication is most effective and least toxic."* These studies also make it possible to administer smaller doses at the most opportune time. As a result, the cost of treatment and the risk of toxicity and side effects can be reduced. It is reasonable to conclude from these studies that awareness of biological rhythms can also increase the efficiency and effectiveness of magnetic treatment.

Man is made of energy, both physical and subtle. The subtle energy is explained by the *chakra* system, and the vital energy by the *tridosha* system. First, let us take a look at the chakra system, which is comprised of seven major chakras.

The seven chakras, located along the spine are spinning disks of subtle energy. This subtle body is superimposed upon our physi-

---

*Translation of an excerpt of *Théma, Encyclopédie Larousse, Sciences de la vie* (Paris: Larousse, 1991).

cal body and can be measured as electromagnetic force (as in Kirlian photography). Each of the chakras governs a specific activity and is associated with a particular gland (or glands), element, color, and so forth. When each chakra is fully functioning, the energy circulates in a consistent movement, from the base of the spine upward, and simultaneously from the forehead to the coccyx. This movement of the subtle energy can be described as a vortex, a circular whirling motion of energy, forming a cavity in the center *(sushumna)*. The energy moves from one chakra to another in a "figure 8" pattern. It spins upward counterclockwise, and downward clockwise. These two currents are called respectively *pingla* and *ida*.

The seven chakras are interrelated. If one becomes blocked, the others cannot function fully to bring equanimity to the nervous system. They are all parts of a whole system of circulating energy. Following is a brief description of each chakra and its associations.

> **Sahasrara** (7th chakra): Crown chakra, located on the top of the head, associated with awareness, the pituitary gland, violet, super ether.
>
> **Ajna** (6th chakra): Forehead, intuition, vision, pineal gland, indigo, ether (light).
>
> **Visshudha** (5th chakra): Throat, communication, hypothalamus and thyroid, blue, ether (sound).
>
> **Anahata** (4th chakra): Heart, love and compassion, thymus, green, air.
>
> **Manipura** (3rd chakra): Solar plexus, energy, power, pancreas, adrenals, yellow, fire.
>
> **Svadhisthana** (2nd chakra): Lower abdomen, emotions, sexuality, orange, water.
>
> **Muladhara** (1st chakra): Base of spine (coccyx), survival, grounding, adrenals, red, earth.

Ayurvedic medicine recognizes three biological rhythms or "movements" in the human body. These are collectively referred to as *doshas* (or *tridoshas*), an ancient Sanskrit term that can also be translated as "humors." According to Ayurvedic principles, everything in the physical universe is composed of five basic elements: earth, water, fire, air, and ether. Indian sages established a link between these natural elements and their effect on the human body and identified three fundamental human "constitutions": *kapha, pitta,* and *vata.* They also established a correlation between each of these doshas and the five senses: Kapha is associated with the elements of earth and water and the senses of smell and taste; pitta is linked to the element of fire and the sense of sight; and vata is connected to the elements of air and ether and the senses of touch and hearing.

Kapha creates vital energy. It plays a role in reproduction, the hydration and lubrication of the body and joints, fat regulation, the shaping of body structures, and protection against disease and aging. According to Dr. Bagwan Dash (who once was the official Ayurveda expert for the government of India), this dosha is located in the gastrointestinal system, at the level of the stomach, and controls food absorption. Some of the physiological symptoms associated with kapha dysfunction are loss of appetite, indigestion, excessive expectoration or excess mucus (bronchitis, asthma, tuberculosis, excessive salivation), excess fat, goiter, the sensation of heaviness or numbness, heart and skin problems, obesity, inflammation of veins, and anemia.

Pitta utilizes vital energy. It assists with oxidation activities, digestion, metabolic function, thermoregulation, and vision, and it is located in the small intestine, liver, spleen, pancreas, and gall bladder. The main symptoms related to pitta dysfunction are excessive sweating; ulcers of the eyes, throat, and mouth; furuncles; excessive hunger and thirst; fever; diarrhea; skin diseases; neuritis; hepatic symptoms; and bleeding.

Vata is an organically invisible force that controls the distribution of vital energy, and in this respect it is sometimes compared to the invisible forces of gravity and electromagnetism. This dosha is involved in muscle movement (voluntary and involuntary), breathing, the flow of vital fluids such as blood and plasma, and waste elimination. It is associated with nerve impulses such as the transmission of messages from one organ to another and subtle meridian and chakra channels, and it is also closely linked to the sensory organs. Vata is located in the gastrointestinal system, at the level of the large intestine. Symptoms associated with vata dysfunction are digestive disturbances, gas and bloating, circulatory problems, headaches, agitation, insomnia, and random pain difficult to locate.

These three principles are present in all human beings in varying proportions. In each person, each dosha is either balanced, deficient, or overdeveloped. The ratio among the doshas is manifested in each person's character, behavior, emotional makeup, and body build. When kapha, pitta, and vata are in balance, spiritual, mental, and physical health prevails. However, in most cases one of the doshas predominates. For example: When kapha predominates, the person is said to have a kapha constitution. If there are two predominant doshas, the person's constitution is identified as vata-pitta, or vata-kapha, or pitta-kapha. The ideal constitution is vata-pitta-kapha, where the three doshas are in perfect balance with one another.

The predominance of a particular dosha is partly inborn and partly acquired. Many aspects of modern life (stress, bad eating habits, lack of exercise, and negative thinking and behavior) contribute to unbalanced tridoshas. This imbalance interferes with the body's relationship to the five elements (earth, water, fire, air, and ether) and has a negative effect on health and general well-being.

Ayurvedic experts have determined that although the energy of the universe is constant, it manifests itself in different ways at regular intervals throughout the year, and even in the course of the day. They have discovered that there is a cyclical predominance of the characteristics associated with each of the three biological movements—kapha, pitta, and vata—at certain hours of the day; each of these periods is favorable to a certain type of activity and has a specific effect on mood and behavior, with such effects varying in strength throughout the day. Practitioners of Ayurvedic medicine claim that knowledge and respect of these cycles can lead to increased personal awareness, and they recommend that you practice each daily activity at its most advantageous period.

In Ayurveda, each twenty-four-hour cycle is divided into six periods of about four hours each, with one of the three doshas predominant in each period. The daytime hours (from dawn to dusk) are divided into three equal parts, with the first governed by kapha, the second by pitta, and the third by vata; the nighttime hours are similarly divided. Table 7 shows what the cycles will be if the sun rises at six o'clock and sets at six in the evening. Please note that in 40° to 50° latitude areas, like Canada, sunrise and sunset times vary greatly from season to season, which means that daytime and nighttime periods will not necessarily always be equal.

TABLE 7

Time	Dosha
6:00 A.M. to 10:00 A.M.	Kapha
10:00 A.M. to 2:00 P.M.	Pitta
2:00 P.M. to 6:00 P.M.	Vata
6:00 P.M. to 10:00 P.M.	Kapha
10:00 P.M. to 2:00 A.M.	Pitta
2:00 A.M. to 6:00 A.M.	Vata

In general, the period governed by kapha is characterized by calm, stability, and consolidation. In contrast, the period dominated by pitta is more dynamic and conducive to activity. The vata period is one of intense creative and mental activity, where mental function tends to be more intuitive than intellectual; it can also be a time of serenity and inspiration.

Each organ has its own rhythm, meaning that it has recurring periods of activity, transition, and recovery that follow logical patterns. Each organ functions at its highest intensity at a particular time in the biological cycle and functions at a significantly reduced level exactly twelve hours later. By treating an organ (or its corresponding channels, which practitioners of Oriental medicine call meridians, or *marmas* in Sanskrit) at the optimal time, the treatment (be it medication, massage, acupuncture, homeopathy, or magnet therapy) will naturally be more effective. However, it is not always practical to treat an organ during its most intense period of activity. For example, the optimal treatment period for the bladder is between three and five o'clock in the afternoon, but the optimal period for the liver is between one and three o'clock in the morning!

In each twenty-four-hour cycle, all organs and viscera have a period of optimal activity that lasts about two hours and a period of minimal activity that occurs twelve hours later. The study of acupuncture has established the activity cycle of the twelve major meridians that affect the organs. However, before discussing the results of these studies, we need to briefly describe the fundamental principles of traditional Chinese medicine.

According to Oriental philosophy, energy is the main element of humans and all living beings and is made up of two complementary poles: yin and yang. These two essential energies are opposed, complementary, and interrelated, all at the same time; one does not exist without the other. Yin attracts yang and yang attracts yin, like opposite poles of a magnet. At the same time, yin repels yin and yang repels yang, like the same poles of a magnet. Yin and yang are inseparable; yin controls yang and yang supports yin. "Yin represents matter, that is, the blood flowing through the body; yang flows on the outside of the body, in order to allow it to be active and defend itself from outside harm."* Yin can be compared to negative electric energy and north pole magnetic energy, whereas yang corresponds to positive electric energy and south pole magnetic energy.

Life is a constant struggle to balance yin and yang energies; as we all know, perfect balance is difficult to achieve and maintain. Most of the time there is a constant back-and-forth movement between yin and yang, a natural oscillation that is to be expected and respected. However, illness often occurs when the degree of imbalance is too great, and in extreme cases imbalance can even cause death. In traditional Chinese medicine, illness is believed to be caused by an imbalance between yin and yang, that is, an excess or lack of one or the other.

---

*Translation of an excerpt from Lise Arcand Müller, *L'acupuncture* (Outremont, Québec: Les Éditions Québécor, 1993), 25.

These invisible energies, which are part of all of us, travel through meridians, the numerous channels that form a network extending to all parts of the body. There are twelve major meridians in the body and sixty secondary ones. The two most important meridians—the conception channel and the regulatory channel—are located along the middle axis of the body. Each meridian contains a specific number of points where energy seems to concentrate. These are known as acupuncture points, the specific locations that an acupuncturist stimulates with needles. These points can also be stimulated by massage (such as Ayurvedic massage or shiatsu), heat *(moxa)*, electricity, laser, or magnetism.* It is believed that currents of energy follow various routes, some at deep levels and others close to the surface. This energy sometimes crosses internal organs, and meridians are often given the name of the organ they most affect, although this is not a consistent practice.

According to Oriental philosophy, the viscera (intestines, etc.) are considered part of the yang category, because they transform outside energy into energy that is useful to the body. The organs (heart, liver, etc.) are yin because they regulate, circulate, and purify the blood. Each yin organ has a corresponding yang viscus: The heart is paired with the small intestine, the liver with the gall bladder, the spleen with the stomach, the lungs with the large intestine, the kidneys with the bladder. The pericardium, a membrane surrounding the heart, is said to be linked to the triple burner meridian, although these two are really functions rather than organs. The triple burner, considered yang, facilitates heart and lung functions in the transport of oxygen through the body, as well as spleen and stomach functions in the digestion and absorption of nutritive elements. The pericardium, which is yin, protects the heart.

The twelve meridians are classified in two categories, just like the organs for which they are named. Half are yang (positive or south pole) and half are yin (negative or north pole). Table 8 lists

---

*Certain devices can determine the exact location of these points.

TABLE 8

Meridian/Organ	Peak period	Polarity
Liver	1 A.M. to 3 A.M.	Yin
Lungs	3 A.M. to 5 A.M.	Yin
Large intestine	5 A.M. to 7 A.M.	Yang
Stomach	7 A.M. to 9 A.M.	Yang
Secretion (spleen/pancreas)	9 A.M. to 11 A.M.	Yin
Heart	11 A.M. to 1 P.M.	Yin
Small intestine	1 P.M. to 3 P.M.	Yang
Bladder	3 P.M. to 5 P.M.	Yang
Kidney	5 P.M. to 7 P.M.	Yin
Heart constrictor	7 P.M. to 9 P.M.	Yin
Triple burner	9 P.M. to 11 P.M.	Yang
Gall bladder	11 P.M. to 1 A.M.	Yang
Conception meridian	24 hours	Yin
Regulatory meridian	24 hours	Yang

the twelve major meridians and the two regulatory meridians, the periods of their most intense activity, and their polarity.

We recommend that you choose the best time for treatment, if at all possible. It is also important to remember that certain people are more sensitive to magnetism than others and therefore will respond to its effects quite rapidly. On the other hand, there are those who do not respond to the effects of magnetism right away. This does not mean that the treatment is ineffective. The response depends on the individual as well as the situation.

For example, if the problem is recent, and not serious, the effect of magnets is usually felt in the first moments of treatment. If the illness is of a more serious nature, or if it has developed over the course of years, it may take several weeks or months to see an improvement. In such cases before giving up on magnetic treatment try the same treatment with a stronger magnet. It is possible, even probable, that this will make the effects perceptible. In case of doubt, however, it is advisable to consult an experienced magnet therapist.

POLARITIES IN THE HUMAN BODY

Everything can be classified in terms of yin and yang: positive and negative, south and north, heat and cold, summer and winter. The human body can be divided both horizontally and vertically, and this yin/yang pattern will always be found. If we divide the body at the waist, the upper body (which includes the head, arms, and chest) is considered positive, or yang, and the lower body (which includes the lower abdomen, legs, and feet) is considered negative, or yin. If the division is made along a vertical axis crossing the solar plexus, the right side is considered positive, or yang, and the left side is considered negative, or yin. Similarly, the front of the body is seen as positive, or yang, and the back as negative, or yin.

In laboratory experiments using very sensitive instruments, researchers have been able to measure the surface voltage of different parts of the body. Results show that along the right side of the body, including the right arm and leg, there is positive voltage ranging between 25 and 65 microvolts. On the left side, there is negative voltage of the same intensity. The highest voltage is located around the navel and decreases downward toward the legs. The experiment was conducted on several subjects; figure 23 provides the average measurements obtained.

These experiments confirmed that the right side of the body has a positive energy

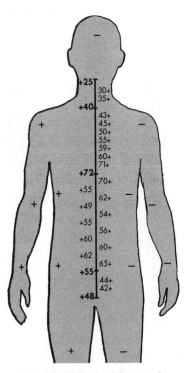

Fig. 23. Voltages Measured on the Human Body

and the left side a negative energy. They identified two points with a high positive charge of about 50 microvolts: the base of the skull (where the neck begins) and the bottom of the spinal column. They also identified two points where there is no charge at all: the point immediately above the first cervical vertebra and the area just below the coccyx, which are the locations where polarity reverses itself. The rest of the spinal column was found to have a negative charge, which is probably because it carries alkaline fluids (alkaline substances are negative and acid substances positive).

The inversion of polarity in the human body is comparable to

TABLE 9

Yang—South—Positive	Yin—North—Negative
Back of the body	Front of the body
Right side	Left side
Upper body	Lower body
Viscera, which receive, digest, and excrete: large intestine, bladder, stomach, gall bladder, small intestines	Organs that produce and store essential elements: heart, lungs, kidneys, liver, spleen

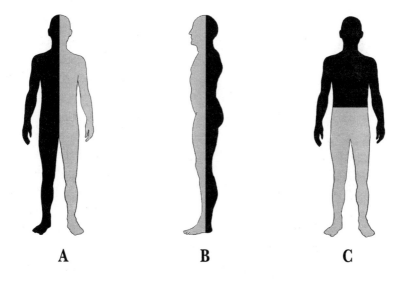

A   B   C

Fig. 24. Polarity of the Body
(A: left side/right side, B: front/back, C: upper/lower half)

85

the energy pattern at the equator, or the figure eight path followed by the lines of force in a straight magnet, as described by Dr. Davis. This energy system is summarized in table 9 and figure 24 for the practical purpose of using magnetism to balance polarity in the human body.

COMBINED THERAPIES

Some practitioners combine the principles of magnetism with other principles, like those used in acupuncture or the Taoist principles of yin and yang. As there are parallels between the north and south magnetic poles, the principles of yin and yang, and negative and positive electric charges, it is probably inevitable that these principles will combine and overlap in practice.

Some experts reinforce the therapeutic effects of acupuncture with magnetism. Others use the meridians of the body to direct magnetic energy through the body as a whole or toward a particular organ. For those familiar with the meridians, it is easy to apply magnetic treatment along these channels. For instance, a small magnet can be applied directly on an acupuncture point and kept in place with adhesive tape for two or three days. This method is less cumbersome than using needles, and just as effective. Of course, optimal results depend on the knowledge and skill of the practitioner.

TREATMENTS

The following treatments all utilize magnetic field energy and are either bipolar or unipolar in nature. We strongly recommend bipolar fields to reestablish metabolic and energetic balance; they also have beneficial effects on acid/base biochemical imbalances caused by inadequate nutrition, MFDS, and most other energy imbalances. We recommend that unipolar fields be used in rare cases only, on small surfaces and for short periods. Ideally, unipolar treatment should be immediately followed by the brief application of a bipolar field, in order to rebalance the polarities.

SLEEPING ON A NORTH-SOUTH AXIS

As indicated earlier, when an iron bar is placed on the earth's north-south axis for a long enough period, the bar becomes bipolar; in other words, it becomes a magnet, albeit a low-intensity one. The same is true of the human body, to a lesser degree. For that reason, it is best to sleep every night with the head northward and the feet pointing south; this practice facilitates regeneration by "recharging our batteries."

Some people are more sensitive to energy fields than others, particularly to the electromagnetic fields produced by electric equipment. These people should not place electric alarm clocks, clock radios, and electric blankets (or any other device that produces an electromagnetic field) near their bed, as some of these devices produce an electromagnetic field even when they are not turned on.* The most frequent health problems experienced by people sensitive to electromagnetic fields (especially older people, or those with weak immune systems) are poor circulation, sleep disturbance, and excess acidity. These effects can be harmful if experienced during the night, because the body is motionless and in a passive state of recovery and therefore more vulnerable. Sometimes changing the position of the bed and removing electric devices is enough to gradually eliminate these effects. If the bed cannot be placed in a north-south axis, an east-west axis should be used (head to the east, feet to the west), an arrangement that follows the direction of the rotation of the earth.

GENERAL COMMENTS ON THE APPLICATION
OF MAGNETIC FIELDS

One of the benefits of magnet therapy is that it allows the body to recharge itself gently. We should not be fooled by the subtle and

---

*A compass allows you to identify the electric devices and outlets that produce significant electromagnetic fields and to see over what distance these fields extend. The compass needle will be deviated by equipment such as computers, water heaters, and electric alarm clocks. The compass allows you to identify a secure zone around the equipment, a zone in which the electromagnetic field is negligible.

delicate effects of this treatment: The magnetic field of the earth is a relatively weak force, and yet it is essential. When astronauts travel in space for extended periods, they suffer the negative effects of being outside the earth's field of gravity. Even on earth, it takes little to either unbalance or recharge the human body. Therefore, it is beneficial for people to expose themselves to the effects of magnetic fields on a regular basis.

To administer magnetic treatment, you need several magnets of various sizes and intensities: two or four strong (2,000-gauss) magnets for general treatment and some types of local treatment, and smaller medium-strength (600-gauss) magnets for local applications. All of your magnets should be easy to handle; a plastic coating makes maintenance easier but is not necessary.

Certain principles should always be followed when administering magnetic treatment; they are outlined in the next four sections.

RELAXATION

Remind the patient throughout the treatment to breathe deeply and slowly and relax both body and mind. Suggest that the patient close his or her eyes during the entire treatment, no matter how long or short. The patient should use this time to rest and obtain

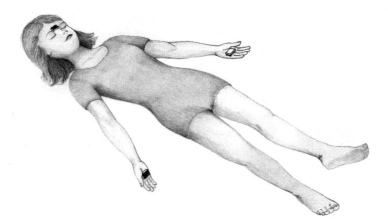

Fig. 25. Treatment in Relaxed Atmosphere

maximum benefit from the magnetic treatment. Make sure the atmosphere of the treatment room is relaxed and that you will not be interrupted. Treatment can be administered while the patient is lying down (head to the north, feet to the south) or comfortably seated.

DURATION AND FREQUENCY OF TREATMENTS

A treatment can last anywhere from five minutes to two hours and can take place anywhere from one to four times a day, as necessary. We recommend that you start with shorter treatments if you do not know how the patient will react to magnetic fields. Be alert for negative reactions such as yawning, a heavy head, prickling sensations, and nausea, as these symptoms could indicate hypersensitivity to magnetic fields. If such symptoms occur, reduce the force of the field and the length of exposure. If the reactions are severe, stop the treatment immediately.

A short treatment should suffice if the problem is relatively recent. However, when the problem has existed for a number of years, several treatment sessions may be necessary. Remember that magnetism is a means of accelerating the healing process, not a cure, and that not all illnesses respond to magnetic treatment.

CHOOSING BETWEEN GENERAL OR LOCAL TREATMENT

A health problem can be local, as in the case of a cut, or general, as in the case of arthritis. Therefore, a magnetic field can be applied to a small surface to treat a specific injury or trauma (in which case the treatment can be either unipolar or bipolar) or to a large surface to provide a more general magnetic effect (in which case the treatment should be bipolar).

COMPATIBILITY WITH OTHER TREATMENTS

Other forms of treatment, such as medication or massage, can be continued along with the application of magnetic fields. Magnet therapy is particularly compatible with homeopathy, acupuncture, and shiatsu. However, when in doubt, you should always check with a doctor to make sure magnetic treatment is compatible with other treatments you or the patient may be receiving. We also recommend you review the "Warnings" section earlier in this chapter on a regular basis to avoid complications.

GENERAL BIPOLAR TREATMENT

This method of magnetic treatment is designed to treat diseases affecting large areas of the body or the entire metabolism of the body. It can also be used to maintain or improve health generally, or as a preventive measure.

If the problem is located in the lower body, the magnets are to be applied to the soles of the feet. If the problem affects the upper body, the magnets are to be placed in the palms of the hands. This treatment always uses both poles in order to close the energy circuit; hence the term "bipolar treatment." The aim is to let the energy flow through the entire body (or a particular portion of the body), but without causing an imbalance. The energy flows between the two magnetic poles and passes through several organs, the meridians, and the blood vessels. For example, when the south pole of a 2,000-gauss magnet is placed against the sole of the right foot and the north pole of a similar magnet against the sole of the left foot, the magnetic energy flows between the two poles, and through the lower body and organs.

When a magnet is placed in the open palm of the hand, only the pole directly touching the hand produces an effect. However, if the fingers close over the magnet, it causes the magnetic current to flow in a closed circuit, in which case both poles exert their effects. Therefore, when the intention is to apply unipolar treatment, the fingers of the hand must remain open in order to achieve the unipolar effect.

RECOMMENDED METHODS

Because the right side of the body is yang, or active, and the left side is yin, or passive, we generally recommend the use of the south pole on the right side and the north pole on the left side, especially in bipolar treatment.

For bipolar treatments, we suggest the use of two flat magnets having a large surface area, as this type of magnet has greater penetration power. The magnetic field of a large-area magnet is wider than that of a smaller magnet of the same intensity. The magnets used should be between 2,000 gauss and 3,000 gauss on the surface. Normally, a general treatment lasts between ten and thirty minutes and can be repeated two or three times a day; however, this type of treatment should never be given for more than an hour per day, because the magnets used are rather strong and overstimulation is not desirable.

The treatments we recommend are like those described by Dr. Bansal, who recommends the application of positive energy to the palm of the right hand and negative energy to the palm of the left hand. However, please note that Dr. Bansal calls the positive pole where induction lines emerge "north pole," whereas we use the opposite designation. Because of this, reading his book* may cause confusion. However, the theories and applications are the same, and it is only the polar terms that differ.

Magnets should be applied according to the methods described in table 10 and figure 26 A and B. We especially recommend methods A and B, which have given very effective results over a number of years.

TABLE 10: RECOMMENDED METHODS FOR MAGNET PLACEMENT

Method A	South pole	Right hand
	North pole	Left hand
Method B	South pole	Right foot
	North pole	Left foot
Method C	South pole	Left hand
	North pole	Left foot
Method D	South pole	Right hand
	North pole	Right foot

*R. S. Bansal and H. L. Bansal, *Magneto Therapy, Self-Help Book* (New Delhi, India: B. Jain Publishers PVT Ltd., 1989).

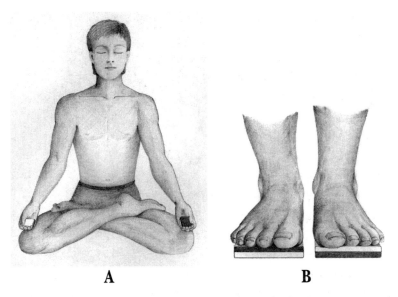

A   **B**

Fig. 26. Placement of Magnets for General Bipolar Treatment:
Methods A and B

Method A (right-hand/south and left-hand/north) creates a magnetic circuit in the upper body. The current affects the chest cavity and the organs it encloses. According to chronobiological principles, the best time to apply this treatment for lung relief is between three and five o'clock in the morning.

Method B (right-foot/south and left-foot/north) is useful for problems located in the lower body, legs, and feet; it also helps to activate the kidneys and relieve urinary problems. Applying the south pole to the right foot and the north pole to the left foot stimulates energy flow in all of the organs below the navel. This method is particularly useful for treating urinary problems and is optimally used between three and five o'clock in the afternoon (for the bladder) and between five and seven o'clock in the evening (for the kidneys).

Method C (left-hand/south and left-foot/north) creates a strong magnetic current that reinforces the energy of the organs and meridians on the left side of the body. Stomach problems should be treated between seven and nine o'clock in the morning.

Method D (right-hand/south and right-foot/north) is best for problems located on that side. With this method, the energy flows through the meridians and organs located on that side. Liver and portal vein problems are best treated between one and three o'clock in the morning.

THE MAGNETIC BELT

We recommend the use of a magnetic belt, the effectiveness of which has been demonstrated over and over again. A magnetic belt is a strip of material made of natural fiber—preferably cotton, silk, or wool—with little pockets in which to insert magnets. Depending on the size of the person, six to ten or even more magnets can be inserted, with polarities alternating. If you make the belt yourself, we suggest you include Velcro strips to allow for easy adjustment of the belt's size. Make sure you remove the magnets before washing.

The magnetic belt functions in two ways: It can be used to correct a specific health problem, and it can be used to generally maintain optimal health. For the latter purpose, the magnets in the belt should be approximately 500 gauss each; one magnet with north polarity should be placed in the middle of the front portion of the belt (near the navel); and, because

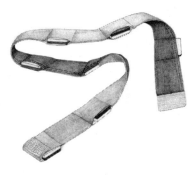

Fig. 27. Magnetic Belt

polarities are alternated, there should be an equal number of north and south polarities. Remember that magnets should never be in direct contact with the spine; they can be placed on either side of the spine, but never directly on it.

When magnets are used to correct a specific health problem, it is best to consult an experienced magnetotherapist who is qualified to determine the number of magnets to be used, as well as their strength, polarity, and placement. The number of magnets might be even or odd, or greater or less than 500 gauss, depending on the condition. The therapist should also determine the material of the belt, where it should be placed, and how long it should be worn.

A magnetic belt is usually worn around the waist to reinforce the digestive system and urinary tract, as well as to relieve a variety of abdominal problems, such as constipation, menstrual pain, and prostate conditions. However, it can also be worn around an arm or a leg to relieve muscular pain due to tension in the upper back, neck, and shoulders. For shoulder and neck pain, the belt can be replaced by a magnetic necklace made of magnetized beads, which is more attractive.

LOCAL UNIPOLAR AND BIPOLAR TREATMENT

Some kinds of pain are very localized, such as pain in the throat or the pain resulting from closing a car door on your finger. In these cases, the magnet should be applied either directly to the affected area or on the meridian connected with the area. Local treatment can always be reinforced by general treatment.

Local treatment uses magnets between 500 gauss and 2,000 gauss. If you do not know how the person you are treating reacts to magnetism, start with 500- to 600-gauss magnets, for short periods of about twenty minutes. If there are no negative effects, increase the strength of the magnets little by little, and use them for gradually longer periods. Such magnets can be applied for several hours with no danger, and the treatment can be repeated three or four times a day. However, if there is no improvement after five days, magnetic treatment should be stopped and the patient should consult a doctor.

Local treatment can be either bipolar or unipolar. Unipolar local treatment applies the north pole of a magnet directly to the painful area. The treatment should last a minimum of fifteen minutes and a maximum of two hours. Bipolar local treatment uses two magnets, one on each side of the affected area. For instance, in the case of a sore knee, the north pole is to be placed on the sore area of the knee and the south pole behind the knee in the exact opposite spot. The magnetic current will then flow precisely where it is needed. If the pain covers a larger area, such as a thigh, two or three magnets (north pole) are to be applied to the painful area and the same number of magnets (south pole) to the area opposite.

The following sections list benign problems that can be treated at home with the application of magnets. Be sure to choose the right method, and consult the corresponding figures.

HEADACHES

Headaches have various causes and can be located in different areas: the forehead, the temples, or the back of the head. Of course, if the exact cause of the headache is known (such as bad digestion) the treatment will be more effective because the magnets can be applied directly to the source of the problem. However, if the cause of the headache is not known, the pain can be eased by treating the area where it is felt. For the head, medium-strength magnets are best (about 500 gauss). Please note that the south pole should never be applied alone to the head.

Depending on the location of the pain, one magnet is to be applied to the right temple and another magnet, with the opposite pole, to the left temple for ten minutes. If only one magnet is used, the north pole is to be applied to the forehead, between the eyebrows. This method produces calm and concentration. Many people use this method when

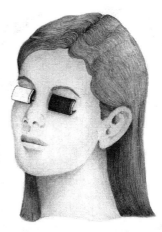

Fig. 28. Magnets on the Eyes (south/right and north/left)

they meditate and report that it has beneficial effects. Small magnets can also be used to relieve tired eyes, with the north pole applied to the left eye and the south pole to the right eye (see figure 28).

Stress often causes stiffness of the neck and sometimes headaches as well. If this is the case, small magnets can be applied to the back of the neck for about ten minutes, on each side of the spine, using the south pole on the right and the north pole on the left. Unipolar treatment can also be applied, using only north poles to ease the pain. Before applying the magnets, the neck and shoulder muscles should be massaged to stimulate blood circulation and promote relaxation. It also helps if the patient does relaxation exercises beforehand, such as rolling the shoulder muscles forward and backward. If such stress headaches are frequent, the patient would also benefit from exercises that strengthen the neck muscles.

PAIN

Pain can be nervous or muscular in origin. When it is clear that the pain is muscular and not due to infection, the south pole can be applied directly to the painful area. The south pole facilitates muscle relaxation and eases this kind of pain. However, it is very important to make sure that no source of infection is present, as the south pole can stimulate growth in general, including that of germs and bacteria, and that is definitely not desired! If you are dealing with nervous pain or pain of unknown origin, the north pole only should be used. In these cases, there are no precautions to be taken other than those listed at the beginning of this chapter.

Toothaches often come on suddenly, and you might not be able to see a dentist right away. Rather than just waiting and suffering, try applying the north pole of a 600- to 2,000-gauss magnet directly to the painful area. Do this as often as needed to relieve the pain while you're waiting to see your dentist. If you have an abscess, use of the north pole is strongly recommended, especially since the abscess has to subside before a dentist can start treatment. To reduce infection, drink north-magnetized water and rinse your mouth with the water several times a day.

JOINT PAIN

Joint pain is very bothersome, whether it involves the elbows, knees, fingers, or shoulders. When such pain persists, people wish for nothing more than the pain to disappear. Fortunately, this is not at all hard to achieve. Simply apply one magnet with the north pole on the painful side of the joint and another one with the south pole on the opposite side (see figure 29).

Generalized joint pain is sometimes caused by MFDS or rheumatism. In these cases, magnets should be applied to the whole body rather than to one restricted area. It is also helpful to drink magnetized water on a regular basis. (The preparation and benefits of magnetized water are discussed in the next chapter.)

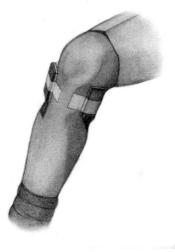

Fig. 29. Treatment of the Joints

Shooting pain in the legs often involves the sciatic nerve, which causes pain to radiate along the entire length of the leg. This kind of pain in the legs and arms requires bipolar magnet application, with the north pole on one side of the affected extremity and the south pole on the opposite side. The number of magnets used depends on the surface involved. It is important to cover the whole area with magnets placed 5 to 10 cm apart. Treatment should last about ten minutes and can be repeated three or four times a day.

INFECTIONS

In the case of infection, the north pole is placed directly on the infected area for about ten minutes twice a day. It is also beneficial to wash skin infections, such as acne, with north magnetized water. Drinking six to eight glasses of magnetized water a day will also help to eliminate toxins and enhance health.

ASTHMA

People suffering from asthma benefit from both local and general treatment. The local treatment involves the application of magnets to the shoulder blades. However, because the heart is near this area, it is important to use medium-strength magnets only, and to be wary of any possible adverse effects. This treatment should be reinforced by the daily application of Method A discussed in the Recommended Methods section (south pole in the right palm and north pole in the left palm). If an asthma attack subsequently occurs, a second general treatment session should be given. It is also helpful for the patient to drink mixed magnetized water several times a day (see chapter 6).

PAINFUL MENSTRUATION

Many women complain of painful menstruation, which is often related to problems of elimination, particularly constipation. Therefore, we recommend that women who suffer from this complaint drink mixed magnetized water on a regular basis and maintain a diet high in fiber, especially on the days preceding the onset of menstruation. Normally, these measures will cause the pain to diminish or completely disappear. However, if the pain persists and medical exams have revealed no pathology, Method B (south pole under right foot, north pole under left foot) should be applied. Local use of the north or south pole depends on the presence or absence of infection; when in doubt the north pole only should be used. Wearing a magnetic belt can also be beneficial.

FEVER

Fever is a defense reaction that is activated when the body has to fight toxins, germs, and waste. Fever is beneficial and, unless life threatening, it should not be impeded. If the fever process is interrupted, the offending germs and toxins in the body will only multiply and increase, causing further damage. On the first day of a fever, this defense mechanism should be allowed to run its course; however, the patient can assist the elimination of toxins by drinking large quantities of north magnetized water and eating as little as possible. It is also important to watch for signs of constipation. The discomfort of a fever can be alleviated with cold compresses on the temples and forehead and the arms and legs. However, if the fever persists or appears life threatening, a doctor should be consulted in order to determine and treat the cause.

MAGNETIC OBJECTS AVAILABLE ON THE MARKET

Almost all hardware stores sell magnets. They are also sold by school-supply retailers who carry science materials. Magnets come in many different sizes, strengths, and forms. Some magnets are coated with a layer of plastic that helps protect them and make maintenance easier; this is an advantage for those who use their magnets frequently or use them on many people. However, if you use the magnets on yourself only, the plastic coating is not important.

The size and shape of the magnet should be appropriate to the use for which it is intended. For example, it is best to apply small, curved magnets to the eyes, because they are the most comfortable. Also, when magnets are used for massage, they should be big enough to be held firmly in the hand.

Books on magnet therapy mention products imported from various countries. We will give you the names under which those products are distributed in North America, as well as their characteristics. However, bear in mind that although the advertised name of a product may be appealing, usually an ordinary magnet purchased at a hardware store will do just as well, if not better. For

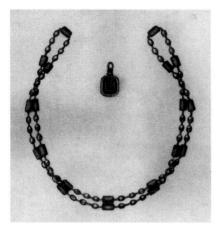

Fig. 30. Magnet Necklace

example, Larry Johnson recommends Yama magnets, which are rectangular 3 cm x 5 cm magnets made in Switzerland, and Marah-Cosam magnets, which are a little smaller than Yama magnets and made of samarium and cobalt. However, the exact strength of Marah-Cosam magnets is not known, so they may not be effective enough for the use intended.

Several authors recommend Biomagnets for application to acupuncture points. These very small 600-gauss magnets (about the size of a pea) are made of barium ferrite and are usually attached to hypoallergenic adhesive tape. They are easy to use in this form, but they can be hard to find. Other magnets of this size are more readily available; they resemble small stars, but do not have adhesive-tape backing.

There are many other products on the market that incorporate magnets for therapeutic purposes, such as mattresses, shoes, knee guards, necklaces, and magnetic belts. However, the polarity and strength of the magnets in these products are not always specified, so there is no way to evaluate beforehand the manufacturer's claims about a product's effectiveness.

Chapter Six

MAGNETIZED WATER

Magnetized water has been used all over world for many years. It is such an important and beneficial form of magnetic treatment that it needs its own chapter!

We will begin by explaining how magnetism acts on water. (Although water does not appear to react to magnetism as dramatically as iron and other materials, it is in fact significantly affected by exposure to magnetic fields.) We will then examine the properties of magnetized water and its effect on plants, animals, and humans. And finally we will explain how to produce this amazing liquid with little effort and cost.

Before discussing the properties of magnetized water, it is necessary to explain certain terms: "North water" refers to water magnetized by the north pole of a magnet; "south water" refers to water magnetized by the south pole of a magnet; and "mixed water" refers to water magnetized by both poles. "Polarized water" is simply another general term for magnetized water, whether unipolar or mixed.

PROPERTIES OF MAGNETIZED WATER

General laboratory tests (such as chemical analyses, pH tests to determine acidity or alkalinity, and mineral content tests) do not detect any changes in water after it has been magnetized. This is why some scientists do not recognize the special properties of magnetized water. However, Dr. Davis spent many years finding ways to demonstrate how water is transformed by exposure to magnetic fields, and he finally succeeded in the early 1970s. He published his research results in *Anatomy of Biomagnetics* in 1974, and other researchers later confirmed and completed his findings.

Research has shown that the following phenomena can be observed after water has been magnetized:

1) increase in hydrogen ion activity

2) decrease in water weight

3) no change in mineral concentrations

4) decrease in quantity of nitrogen dissolved in water

5) increase in the number of crystallization centers

INCREASE IN HYDROGEN ION ACTIVITY

After spending several years researching the properties of magnetized water, the teams of Davis and Rawls observed that the oxygen level of water appeared to drop after magnetization. However, they later realized that it was not the oxygen level that decreased but the hydrogen ion activity that increased. They subsequently performed hundreds of additional experiments that confirmed this finding.

DECREASE IN WATER WEIGHT

Japanese researchers have noted a decrease in the weight of magnetized fluids, particularly water. However, the cause and significance of this decrease is still unknown.

UNCHANGED MINERAL CONCENTRATIONS

Magnetized water has the same beneficial concentration of sodium and calcium as nonmagnetized water, and therefore it is good to drink.

DECREASE IN NITROGEN DISSOLVED IN WATER

Research shows that magnetization reduces the quantity of nitro-gen dissolved in water. Nitrogen accumulates in stagnant or stored water, making it unfit for consumption by humans and aquatic animals. Algae grow in stagnant water by using up the oxygen normally needed by fish, causing millions of fish to die. Because magnetized water reduces nitrogen quantities, it could be used to fight the microorganism invasion or algae overabundance re-sponsible for the disappearance of certain species of fish. It could also be used to maintain the quality of commercial bottled water.

Scientists have discovered that the application of a very strong magnetic field for a very short period (no more than a millisec-ond) has a decontaminating effect: It destroys microorganisms or renders them inactive. This discovery has now been put to practi-cal use in Bordeaux, France, where pulsating magnetic fields are used to sterilize produce. It is logical to deduce that if this proce-dure is effective in decontaminating produce, it would be equally effective on water.

INCREASE IN NUMBER OF CRYSTALLIZATION CENTERS

Research has also proven that exposure to magnetic fields in-creases the number of crystallization centers in liquids. Normally water molecules tend to assemble around foreign particles (usu-ally mineral), which prevents those particles from gathering to-gether to form nucleoli. Although the natural magnetic forces acting on a cluster of water molecules surrounding a particle are very weak, their frequency sometimes coincides with that of the cluster and breaks it up. The liberated particle then attaches itself to other particles, and they assemble to form nucleoli. The advan-tage of these assembled minerals is that they do not form a deposit on the inside surfaces of water pipes.

The term "hard water" is often used to refer to water that reduces the effectiveness of laundry soap or causes deposits to form in the plumbing. One method of softening water and reduc-ing sediment deposits is a difficult and time-consuming process called unplugging. Chemical intervention is the most popular method, but it can cause other problems. Both of these procedures are rather expensive, and have to be repeated regularly.

Fortunately, the application of magnetic fields is a safe and inexpensive alternative method for the treatment and prevention of deposits in water pipes. When water is passed through a magnetic field, the calcium carbonate in the water is modified; it becomes electrically neutral and remains in suspension in the water. The magnetized water dissolves deposits while flowing through the pipes.

This method has been proven effective by thousands of private and commercial users. An article in the French magazine *Science et vie* quotes one of its readers: "Tired of unblocking the 300 m piping of a well with great quantities of chlorine bleach every year, I installed two very strong magnets given to me by a friend. For the past five years I have had no problems."* Another man, the owner of a restaurant, reports that in the two years since he has been using magnetized water there have been no deposits in dishwashers, coffee machines, or toilets. Moreover, he is convinced his coffeepots will last longer and his hot-water costs have been reduced. However, it must be kept in mind that the effects of magnetized water are not instant; it takes six weeks to six months of use before results become apparent.

Water magnetization systems can be installed quickly and easily. They also consume very little electricity and are less expensive than conventional methods of maintaining water quality. As early as the 1950s, countries with minimally developed chemical industries, such as Russia, Poland, Bulgaria, and China, were using this magnetism-based technology. In these countries, magnetism has been used not only in private homes, but also in the treatment of industrial water and in irrigation. Although they at first did not know the reasons for the benefits of magnetized water (e.g., better taste, faster drying), that did not stop them from using it to their advantage.

Science et vie 956 (May 1997):6.

Researchers have also discovered that concrete made with magnetized water is 25 to 35 percent stronger than regular concrete. The reason for this is still unknown, but this discovery will make it possible to produce a lighter and therefore less expensive concrete.

Now that we have seen how magnetism changes the properties of water, we can look at the effect magnetized water has on living beings.

EFFECTS OF MAGNETIZED WATER ON PLANTS

With a little patience, you can conduct your own experiments with plants and magnetized water. Take four identical plants, and for several days water the first with north water, the second with mixed water, the third with south water, and the last with ordinary water. Make sure all of the plants are exposed to the same conditions and environment—light, temperature, humidity, and so on—and do not use fertilizers, which could affect the results. After a

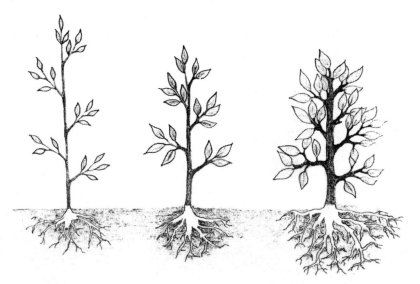

Fig. 31. North water: long, thin plant, sparse foliage; control plant: average height and foliage; south water: short, dense plant, many roots, abundant foliage

few weeks, you will see a significant difference between the plants: North water limits plant growth, producing plants that are taller than normal but rather sparse (like plants that do not receive enough light). Compared with control plants (those given ordinary water), plants that have received south water are shorter, but develop more roots and produce an abundance of leaves, flowers, and fruit.

South water should be used only on the roots of a plant as it stimulates activity exactly where it is used. Using south water on the leaves of a plant could overstimulate the plant in a harmful way. Roots treated with south water already produce abundant foliage, flowers, and fruit, and the plant might not be able to sustain additional leaf growth. Of course, all parts of the plant can be watered with mixed water to generally improve its health, stimulate growth, and prevent disease.

EFFECTS OF MAGNETIZED WATER ON ANIMALS

Most scientific experiments are conducted on animals before they're conducted on human beings, and experiments involving magnetized water are no exception. In Israel, an experimental device that produced magnetized salt water was tested in the dairy industry. After three years of use, the following unexpectedly resulted: The eighty-five cows that drank the magnetized water regularly produced one extra liter of milk per day and were productive a greater number of days, and because they were healthier and stronger, they conceived more easily. Their calves weighed more at birth and were also leaner. To validate these observations, a control group was used. The "magnetized" cows were healthier and more productive than those receiving the usual hormones.

Similar results were obtained with sheep, which produced a better yield of meat, milk, and wool; with chickens and turkeys, which produced more eggs over a longer period; and with geese, which became fatter. Magnetized water has also been tested on lethargic animals in laboratory settings, which within a short time became more active, playful, and interested in their surroundings. It is logical to believe that if magnetized water can have these proven beneficial effects on plants and animals, it must have similar effects on humans.

EFFECTS OF MAGNETIZED WATER ON HUMAN BEINGS

The beneficial effects of magnetized water on human beings are indisputable. Research has proven that magnetized water can improve the digestive system, regenerate tissue, facilitate the elimination of wastes and toxins, strengthen the immune system, and reduce cholesterol.

BENEFICIAL EFFECTS ON THE DIGESTIVE SYSTEM

According to Professor Israel Lin of Technion—Israel Institute of Technology, because magnetized water increases mineral solubility, it improves the distribution of nutrients throughout the body, so that overall body functioning is enhanced. For many years, practitioners in India, Japan, Russia, and other countries have used magnetized water to successfully treat illness, reestablish metabolic balance, and improve the general vitality of otherwise healthy people.

Holger Hanneman advises that the daily consumption of magnetized water is an excellent treatment for constipation and that it should be used in addition to the high-fiber diet that is essential to activate intestines.

REGENERATION OF TISSUES

Magnetized water has special properties that are transferred to the organs of the body after its absorption. The human body is about 70 percent water, so it is very important to replace eliminated water with the best-quality water possible. Blood is also 49.5 percent water. Its function is to supply the body's tissues with the oxygen and nutrients they need and to carry away excess waste—which is another reason we should give our bodies the best water possible.

Drinking magnetized water on a regular basis over a long period not only eliminates digestive problems and acts as a preventive, but it also helps to regenerate tissue. In Puerto Rico, laboratory results (which were later confirmed in a clinical setting with patients) indicated that washing with north water once a day for periods ranging from a few days to two weeks significantly reduced and promoted the healing of bed sores. And patients who subsequently continued this routine did not experience a recurrence of sores.

FACILITATING THE ELIMINATION OF TOXINS

Mixed magnetized water has been shown to improve the body's ability to eliminate toxins. It also improves digestion, reduces gastric acid and flatulence, acts as a diuretic, and has beneficial effects on the urinary system. Holger Hanneman suggests that the daily consumption of a liter of magnetized water is the best way to continue eliminating toxins efficiently. Many people have noticed that it cures constipation in a nonaggressive manner, with no side effects.

In his book *Les aimants pour votre santé* (Magnets For Your Health), Dr. Louis Donnet writes:

In a Leningrad clinic, kidney and bladder stones were dissolved after a course of treatment with magnetized water. However, this water has to be consumed regularly, over a long enough period (two to three months). The magnetic energy it transfers to a living being acts on the entire body. The magnetic field has a positive influence on biological processes. Magnetized water is not a cure in itself but, in conjunction with other forms of treatment, has a synergetic effect. It is diuretic (increases urinary secretion), and stimulates emptying function (allows evacuation of wastes through the organs, such as the kidneys, the lungs, the liver, the pores). The size of the liver is reduced, the bladder becomes less rigid, and there is less pain; small kidney and bladder stones disappear completely within three months. Only urinary calculi remain."*

---

*Louis Donnet, *Les aimants pour votre santé* (St-Jean-de-Braye, France: Éditions Dangles).

In cases of problematic urine elimination, the ingestion of small quantities of magnetized water (about 50 ml) every ten minutes, eight to ten times, has proven very effective for most people. Dr. Bansal also mentions the effective elimination of kidney and bladder stones through the use of magnetized water.

STRENGTHENING THE IMMUNE SYSTEM

Mixed magnetized water generally strengthens the immune system and has proven useful in the treatment of viral infections such as colds, flu, and coughs, as well as conditions like asthma and many other illnesses. Drinking magnetized water on a regular basis has also been shown to generally help the healing process.

REDUCTION OF CHOLESTEROL

Magnetized water has a positive effect on the overall circulation of blood, which, as we mentioned, is almost 50 percent water. The regular consumption of mixed magnetized water has been shown to normalize cholesterol levels; it also prevents the buildup of cholesterol in the arteries and hardening of the arteries, which can lead to high blood pressure, and helps to maintain and regulate heart function.

As we can see, magnetized water is beneficial in so many ways. When magnetized water is consumed regularly over long enough periods, it is both a treatment and a preventive; it improves digestion, facilitates elimination, reduces constipation, has a diuretic effect, dissolves urinary stones, and reduces the severity of menstrual problems. And because it strengthens the immune system, is very useful in the treatment of viral infections such as colds and flu.

NATURALLY MAGNETIZED WATER

Given that water constitutes about 70 percent of the body's weight and is completely replaced every fifteen days, the importance of consuming sufficient amounts of quality water cannot be overemphasized. Water is essential to the proper functioning of the body's metabolism: It ensures the effective transport of elements necessary to the operation and maintenance of the organism and carries out the elimination of waste.

When one speaks of "quality water," many people probably think of spas, and it is very likely that the waters of famous spas are, in fact, naturally magnetized. We know that thermal springs are warm mineral springs originating from inside the earth. In addition to absorbing the heat of the earth's interior, subterranean waters are recharged by magnetic stones, which give them their mineral content. Once they reach the surface, they are recharged again by solar energy. In short, they are constantly being revitalized, which is probably what gives these waters their therapeutic qualities.

Natural spa and spring waters are used for drinking and bathing. They are also used to treat liver, bladder, stomach, and intestinal ailments; exotic diseases; certain kidney conditions; diabetes; urinary tract ailments; and cardiovascular, digestive, and nutritional problems.

LINEUP FOR MIRACLE WATER

An article in the *Washington Post* reports that a man in the Mexican town of Tlacote discovered water on his property that is lighter than tap water and has proven effective in the treatment of AIDS, cancer, obesity, and high cholesterol. Thousands of people who have used this miracle water, which the man dispenses free of charge, claim that it has helped them. Experts say the water is normal for the region, except that it is lighter than normal water, for reasons they cannot explain. Could this be naturally magnetized water?

MAGNETIZED WATER AT HOME

Unfortunately, most of us do not have access to the benefits of these faraway and expensive sources of therapeutic waters. Although approved by our governments, our own water systems are chemically treated and sometimes polluted by toxic agents.

We need good-quality water to maintain the best health possible.

So why not use magnetic fields to revitalize the water that is available to us?

THE USES OF MAGNETIZED WATER

Magnetized water is usually taken internally, but it can also be used externally to clean the eyes, bathe a wound, or reduce the pain of a burn and prevent blistering. We have also seen that the direct application of north water is beneficial in the treatment and prevention of bed sores.

Many users say that tap water tastes and smells better after it has been magnetized. Few of us have access to pure spring water from a clean well; and if we cannot buy bottled water or use a water purifier, we must drink chemically treated tap water, which has a smell some people find intolerable. According to Dr. Klaus Kronenberg, a scientist who has studied in the United States and Germany, this odor is produced by sulfate particles dissolved in the water. When water is magnetized, these particles are solidified, and their odor goes away.

The many advantages of using magnetized water cannot be disputed. However, we are pleased to report that magnetized water is also easy and inexpensive to produce.

PREPARING MAGNETIZED WATER

Unipolar Water: North Water and South Water

Magnetizing water is relatively easy. Simply fill a glass container* with tap water and place the container on a high-strength flat magnet (about 1,000 gauss). Experts disagree about the amount of time required for magnetization, but the average time recommended is between twelve and twenty-four hours. The time required is the same for both mixed and unipolar water.

---

*A plastic container can also be used. However, because plastic has a petroleum base and keeps odors longer, we recommend the use of a glass container.

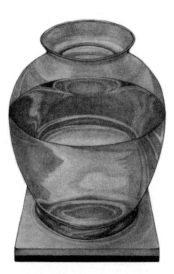

*Fig. 32. Method for Obtaining
North-Magnetized Water*

Dr. Davis recommends that the container be left on the magnet permanently, and that it be regularly refilled as the water is consumed. One simple method is to fill a pitcher of water every night and leave it on magnets until morning. The next day you have magnetized water; that evening, start over again.

North or south water is produced depending on the pole of the magnet used. Magnets should never be dipped in water, because they can rust. They can be used outside the container, however, since magnetism goes through plastic or glass. The magnets used to magnetize the water should be placed on a paramagnetic material, such as wood. They should not be placed near metal objects, such as a toaster or refrigerator, because that may cause demagnetization.

Water magnetized in this way will keep its properties for a maximum of three days. Ideally, magnetized water should be stored at room temperature, because cold liquids can cause stomach cramps. However, you can keep the water in the refrigerator if the shelves are made of glass and not of metal, and as long as you place the container in the center of the refrigerator, away from the metallic walls and any other metallic objects, such as utensils, tins, jar lids, and so forth.

Mixed Water

In Russia, magnetized water is produced by dripping water slowly between the two poles of a U-shaped magnet. Although magnetized water produced in this way has both polarities, the method is not very practical. A simpler method is to lay flat magnets side by side, in a checkerboard pattern, as shown in figure 33.

The magnets will naturally attract and form a stand; by placing a container of water on this stand, you will obtain water that has both north and south magnetization. This is one of the easiest ways to produce mixed water at home.

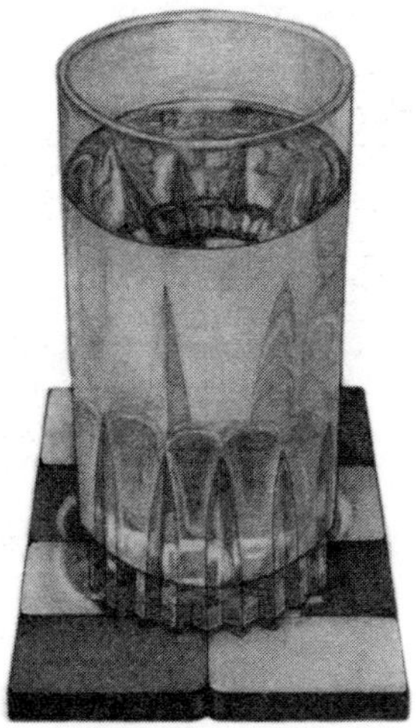

Another simple method is to place a liter of water on the north end of a strong magnet and another liter on the south end of an equally strong magnet. After a few hours, mix the water in the two containers together. This will produce two liters of mixed magnetized water.

Fig. 33. Method for Obtaining Mixed Water

You can also buy electric devices that produce a magnetic field and transmit it to the water. Such devices have been patented since the fifties and have been used for years in Russia, China, Poland, Bulgaria, and other countries. There are now devices on the market in North America that use electromagnets to magnetize water in less than two hours. However, these devices are expensive and not necessarily more effective than permanent magnets.

Regardless of the method of magnetization, magnetized water retains its charge for a period of two to three days, as long as it is kept away from metal objects that could potentially demagnetize it.

DOSES

The body loses a certain amount of water each day. How much water is lost varies from one individual to another, depending on personal habits, but the average is 2,500 ml per day. The method of elimination is as follows: 60 percent in the urine, 28 percent through the skin and the lungs, 8 percent in sweat, and 4 percent in feces. The daily elimination of toxins also results in loss of water and minerals. When the body is dehydrated, the system has difficulty eliminating toxins and there is a risk of toxification.

To avoid being dehydrated, lost water must be replaced on a regular basis. Water is replaced as follows: 60 percent through drinks ingested, 30 percent by the moisture contained in food, and 10 percent by the body's metabolism. Therefore, a person should drink a liter to a liter and a half of water per day. We cannot overemphasize how essential water is to life.

Generally, the recommended daily intake of mixed water for average-size healthy adults is 250 ml (about 8 oz), six to ten times a day. However, you can start with three glasses and gradually increase the quantity until you reach the suggested maximum, or the amount you can tolerate. We also recommend that you always drink one glass of room temperature magnetized water as soon as you get up, before eating. This helps to clean the colon, promote regularity, strengthen the heart, oxygenate the brain, as well as instill an overall sense of tranquillity and well-being.

Mixed water is used more often than unipolar water, because it generally increases energy levels and resistance in otherwise healthy people. North water has calming effects and is usually taken internally in the case of infections like cold, flu, and throat inflammation; or it can be used externally, for bathing the skin or eyes in case of inflammation. South water is more stimulating and therefore is used more rarely, though it can be very beneficial in the case of general fatigue. However, when in doubt, it is best to use mixed water or north water.

MAGNETIZING OTHER SUBSTANCES

If water can be magnetized, so can other liquids, such as oil and milk. But one must be careful with milk, as it cannot be kept at room temperature for very long; also, the south pole of a magnet tends to cause milk to sour. As for oil, because it is more viscous than water, it should be magnetized for at least fifteen days before use. Magnetized oil is used mostly for massage: A north-magnetized oil produces a calming effect and is recommended for the massage of painful joints, aching muscles, and problem skin. It is also helpful to massage north oil on the scalp for the treatment of insomnia. A massage with south-magnetized oil can be useful in treating weakness, paralysis, and baldness.

Chapter Seven

CASES

At the National Research Institute for Self-Understanding, we have been recommending and monitoring the use of magnets for many years. As a result, we have been able to conduct our own research on the effectiveness of magnet therapy and collect data on its use. This final chapter includes some actual cases of clients and friends of the Institute who have used magnet therapy with positive results. This research is, of course, incomplete; however, the case histories confirm the findings of experts in this area, and we would like to share them with you.

SCIENTIFIC RESEARCH

One of the main criticisms of biomagnetic research is that it is not rigorous enough and does not conform to scientific standards. "It has not been scientifically proven" is a frequent comment. However, we wish to examine what this phrase actually means.

Scientists agree that properly conducted research consists of several stages: research design, implementation, and analysis and interpretation of results. All serious researchers strive to meet these established scientific criteria.

RESEARCH DESIGN

Researchers begin by defining working hypotheses, which they try to confirm through experiment. They then establish research protocols that outline the methods that will be used. No detail of their experiments can be overlooked if they wish to ensure that the validity of results will not be jeopardized.

IMPLEMENTATION

To carry out their experiments, researchers choose participants based on an objective selection technique, and then they divide them into groups (most often two) at random, based on a statistical method. The groups should be similar but not necessarily identical. One of the groups receives the experimental treatment that is the subject of the research and the other acts as a control group and is given a placebo treatment.

Ideally, the research should be double-blind. This means that neither the researchers nor the participants know who is receiving the experimental treatment and who is receiving the placebo. It is important to make sure that all the participants receive or take their treatment.

ANALYSIS AND INTERPRETATION OF RESULTS

When the experiment has been completed, researchers examine the results carefully, using the most precise and objective method of observation possible. They compile and analyze the data. They also submit it to expert statisticians who determine the statistic probability that the differences observed between the two study groups may be due to chance.

Finally, researchers draw their conclusions, which will either confirm or oppose their initial hypotheses, and determine the extent to which the results are statistically significant. A discovery has been "scientifically proven" only when the results have been repeated and reproduced by different scientists in similar but distinct circumstances. If not, the results can be questioned; skeptics can claim that the experimental method lacked objectivity, that the sample did not meet scientific criteria, or that the experiment cannot be reproduced. Although this does not necessarily mean the researchers' conclusions are false, their research must meet these rigorous standards in order to be taken seriously by the scientific community.

Therefore, anyone researching the effects of biomagnetism must be very careful to provide as much information as possible about their experiments so that others can repeat them and compare their results. Please take the time to describe all aspects of your experiments in detail.

However, that being said, it is a fact that important discoveries are often made by chance under very unscientific circumstances. Dr. Davis's accidental discovery in 1936 of the differences between north and south pole effects is a case in point (see chapter 5). Therefore, even though the cases we are presenting in this chapter may not qualify as "scientific," they are nonetheless significant in that they confirm the research results of Davis, Bhattacharya, Bansal, Rawls, Sierra, Hanneman, and other experts who have dedicated years of their lives to the study of biomagnetism.

We should also remember that some individuals are more sensitive to magnetism than others, just as some people can have different reactions and sensitivity to traditional medications and treatments. This can explain why the results of magnetic treatment vary from one case to another, especially in terms of the length of time it may take the patient to respond to the treatment.

RESEARCH REPORT

The research data we have collected at the Institute confirm the healing effects of magnets. The assumptions underlying our recommended treatments and research are as follows: that north and south poles produce different effects; that the north pole (negative) reduces, dissolves, and contracts; and that the south pole (positive) augments and stimulates. The strength of the magnets used varies between 100 and 3,500 gauss, with the weakest used on small areas and the strongest on large surfaces. We have also tested magnetic belts and magnetized water.

In the following case studies, the patients were asked these specific questions:

1) Why did you decide to use magnet therapy?

2) What specific problem did you seek to relieve with magnet therapy?

3) How long did you have this problem before beginning magnet therapy?

4) How long (days, weeks, months) did you use magnet therapy to treat the problem?

5) Where on your body did you apply the magnets?

6) Which pole of the magnet was touching your skin during the treatment?

7) How long did you leave the magnets on?

8) How many times a day did you repeat the treatment?

9) What improvements did you notice, and when?

The cases and collected data were classified according to the following categories: pain, relaxation, general well-being, breathing passages, nervous system, infections, and magnetized water.

PAIN

One of the main benefits of the north pole magnetic field is its ability to reduce pain. When you know the cause of the pain, north pole treatment can be used to decrease a patient's discomfort level while healing and other treatments take effect. However, if you are not sure of the cause, a medical professional should be consulted to ensure the pain is not the symptom of a more serious problem.

Case A, February 1992

S. D. experienced lower back pain. She applied the north pole of a 1,500-gauss magnet to the right side of her back, and after three weeks of continuous use the pain disappeared completely.

Case B, February 1992

At forty years old, F. R. sprained an intercostal muscle on the left side of her chest. She applied eight small 1,000-gauss magnets directly to her skin, with the north pole on the muscle. She wore the magnets twenty-four hours a day for a week, and after five days the pain was gone.

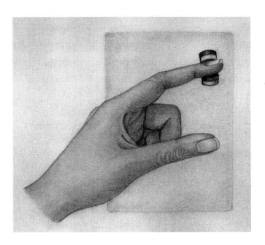

Fig. 34. Magnets on Finger

Case C, April 1992

P. M. had a door slammed on his finger, after which he experienced a throbbing pain and was not able to bend his finger. The north pole of a 1,500-gauss magnet was placed against the nail of the injured finger, and the south pole of an equal-strength magnet was applied to the other side of the finger against the skin. Within five minutes the throbbing pain disappeared.

Case D, September 1992

S. B. reported that the north pole of a 1,500-gauss magnet relieved her headaches and backaches when she applied it for ten minutes or longer.

Case E, March 1993

E. P., a forty-seven-year-old secretary, reported that she used the north pole of a round, 150-gauss magnet to relieve the pain in *her upper back, near her right shoulder. This pain had been so incapacitating that she could not work at her computer for more than half an hour. After wearing the magnet for only two weeks, the pain was reduced by half and she was able to work again.*

For another pain in the lower back, E. P. used four 150-gauss magnets, two on each side, at the bottom of her spinal cord. She applied one north pole and one south pole to each side. She wore the magnets twenty-four hours a day for three and a half months, and as a result the pain disappeared completely and did not return for six months. She now feels a slight recurrence of pain whenever she is stressed or very tired but is able to obtain quick relief as soon as she applies the magnets.

Case F, January 1994

M. suffered from neck and back pain as a result of a car accident several years earlier. She was able to cure this pain in six months by placing the south pole of five 1,200-gauss magnets on her neck and along her spinal cord.

Case G, September 1994

G. R. had a painful bunion on one of his toes. After scraping off the surface of the bunion, he wore a small 1,000-gauss magnet directly on his toe, with the north pole against the skin, six hours a day for a total of three days. After three days, he experienced no more pain.

Case H, October 1994

B. B. experienced pain in her knee. She wore a knee guard equipped with two 1,500-gauss magnets, with one magnet on each side of the knee and the north poles touching the skin. She felt a tingling sensation after only a few minutes, and the pain subsided.

Case I, November 1994

N. succeeded in eliminating the pain of a broken finger in only two nights by applying the north pole of a 200-gauss magnet directly to the finger.

Case J, December 1994

G. N. applied the north pole of a 200-gauss magnet near his kidneys for twenty minutes at a time, several times a day, and the pain he was experiencing in this area eventually disappeared.

Case K, February 1995

K. K., who was experiencing muscle pain in his back, used the north pole of six 200-gauss magnets, three on each side of his spinal cord. He slept with the magnets on at night but did not wear them during the day. After six days, the pain was gone.

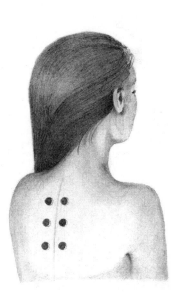

Fig. 35. Magnets on Back

Case L, April 1995

H. D. experienced a burning sensation in her neck. For two weeks she wore a magnetic belt equipped with nine 200-gauss magnets, with the north poles against the skin; she wore it twelve hours a day on weekdays, and twenty hours a day on weekends. This treatment helped ease the tension in her neck and eliminated the burning sensation.

Case M, July 1995

A. M. experienced pain just above her lower back. She wore a magnetic belt equipped with nine 200-gauss magnets, with the north poles against the skin. After only one minute, she no longer felt any pain; however, she continued to wear the belt as a preventive measure for two hours in the morning and two hours in the late afternoon.

TABLE 11: VARIOUS TYPES OF PAIN

Case	Problem	Magnet	Pole	Duration	Observation
A	Lower back pain	One 1,500-gauss magnet	North	Continuously for three weeks	Pain completely disappeared
B	Intercostal muscle sprain	Eight 1,000-gauss magnets	North	Twenty-four hours a day for a week	Pain disappeared after five days
C	Crushed finger	Two 1,500-gauss magnets	North South	Only once, for five minutes	Pain disappeared
D	Headaches Backaches	One 1,500-gauss magnet	North	About ten minutes	Significant relief
E1	Back pain	One 1,500-gauss magnet	North	Two weeks	Pain diminished by half
E2	Back pain	Four 150-gauss magnets	North South	Twenty-four hours a day for three and a half months	Pain completely disappeared
F	Back and neck pain	Five 1,200-gauss magnets	South	Continuously for six months	Relief
G	Bunion on toe	One 1,000-gauss magnet	North	Six hours a day for three days	Pain disappeared after three days
H	Knee	Two 1,500-gauss magnets	North	A few minutes	Tingling sensation followed by almost instant relief
I	Broken finger	One 200-gauss magnet	North		Pain disappeared after two nights
J	Kidney pain	One 200-gauss magnet	North	Periods of twenty minutes several times a day	Pain eventually disappeared
K	Back muscle pain	Six 200-gauss magnets	North	Only during the night	Pain disappeared after six days with three magnets on each side of spinal cord
L	Neck pain	Nine 200-gauss magnets	North	Twelve to twenty hours a day for two weeks	Relief of tension and disappearance of burning sensation
M	Lower back pain	Nine 200-gauss magnets	North	Two hours in the morning, two hours in the late afternoon	Almost instant disappearance of pain

RELAXATION, WELL-BEING, MEDITATION

In *Magnetic Healing and Meditation,* Larry Johnson writes that "meditation, martial arts, and athletic training are areas where regular use of magnets can be beneficial for balancing and reinforcing the effects of these activities."* A number of clients and friends of the Institute have experienced this benefit of magnetism and have shared their observations with us. Whether they used a magnet over the "third eye," wore a magnetic belt, or drank magnetized water, all reported experiencing consequent feelings of calm and well-being.

Case N, February 1992

A 1,500-gauss magnet was placed over S. D.'s thymus gland (on the sternum) during meditation, with the south pole against the skin, to treat her depression. She did this for twenty minutes each morning and evening for one month. She reports that her depression gradually lifted and that she is now able to face whatever life brings her.

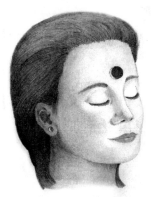

S. D. also applied the north pole of a 1,500-gauss magnet to the sole of her left foot and the south pole of another 1,500-gauss magnet to the sole of her right foot every night while she slept. They were placed at reflexology points corresponding to the solar plexus, and she noticed that this treatment gave her a remarkable feeling of well-being.

Fig. 36. Magnet on Third Eye

Case O, February 1992

F. R. wore a magnetic belt equipped with nine small 200-gauss magnets with north poles against the skin, in an effort to bring more calm and peace to her life.

---

*Larry Johnson, *Magnetic Healing and Meditation* (San Francisco: White Elephant Monastery, 1988).

She did this for one hour each morning and evening, for eight months. This gave her a general sense of well-being and now she uses her belt only when she feels she needs it.

Case P, March 1992

H. L. massaged her temples with a 200-gauss magnet first in a counterclockwise and then in a clockwise direction, also in an effort to bring peace to her life. She used the north pole on her left temple and the south pole on her right temple for ten minutes. This had a very calming effect and she fell peacefully asleep for forty-five minutes. She felt the same calming effect when she rubbed the magnet on her third eye.

Case Q, March 1992

A. T. used a small 2 x 3/4 in. magnet (about 300 gauss) on her third eye to improve her concentration, and she was pleased with the results. She also places her feet on a magnet for twenty minutes a day while reciting the Gayatri mantra, and she reports that this makes her feel stronger and more in balance.

Case R, October 1993

M. R. uses a headband equipped with two 200-gauss magnets, with north poles against the skin. She wears the headband for twenty-five minutes each morning and evening and reports that this gives her a feeling of calm. When her eyes are tired, she applies the north poles of the magnets directly over her eyes for five minutes. M. R. also wears a magnetic belt for two hours each morning and reports that this gives her energy and even prevents flatulence.

Case S, July 1994

S. F. reports that when he places the north pole of a 200-gauss magnet on his forehead during meditation, his concentration immediately improves, and he is better able to focus on the mantra he is reciting.

Case T, August 1994

As a treatment for insomnia, O. S. placed the north pole of a 200-gauss magnet over the middle of his forehead, and he reported that this method proved effective from the first night he used it.

BREATHING PASSAGES

Case U, February 1992

F. R. decided to wear a magnetic belt as a treatment for her asthma. She wore the belt every day for three consecutive hours, and every evening for half an hour, and after two months her condition improved 75 percent. Her asthma disappeared almost entirely, and she now only has to wear the belt once a month to maintain her health.

Case V, March 1992

H. L. had a cold and congested bronchial tubes. She kept the north pole of a 1,500-gauss magnet on each side of her upper chest for ten minutes and then placed it on her throat for five minutes, after which her bronchial congestion disappeared.

TABLE 12: BREATHING PASSAGES

Case	Problem	Magnet	Pole	Duration	Observation
U	Asthma	Nine 200-gauss magnets	North	Three consecutive hours a day and a half hour each evening	75% improvement within two months
V	Bronchial congestion	One 1,500-gauss magnet	North	Ten minutes on each side of chest then five minutes on throat	Relief

THE NERVOUS SYSTEM

Magnets not only help to relieve pain, they also have a beneficial effect on the nervous system, as the following cases illustrate.

Case W, February 1992

At age forty, H. L. developed severe sciatic pain all along her leg. She applied the north pole of a 1,500-gauss magnet on the most painful spot (where the sciatic nerves come together across the buttocks) for ten minutes, and she reported that her pain was subsequently reduced by half.

TABLE 13: THE NERVOUS SYSTEM

Case	Problem	Magnet	Pole	Duration	Observation
W	Sciatic pain	One 1,500-gauss magnet	North	Ten minutes	50% improvement
X	Trembling of hands and feet	Two 1,500-gauss magnets	North South	Five to ten minutes several times a day	Complete relief after twenty days of treatment
Y	Nervous problems	Nine 200-gauss magnets	South	One hour morning and evening	Treatment was successful

Case X, September 1992

At age sixty-three, S. B. began to experience trembling in her hands and feet. She thought she was suffering from Parkinson's Disease, but a medical exam ruled that diagnosis out and her doctor could find no cause for her tremors. S. B. decided to place two 1,500-gauss magnets, one with the north pole side and the other with the south pole side, on different spots on her body for five- to ten-minute periods. She also applied them to the soles of her feet and to reflexology points corresponding to the pancreas and the kidneys several times a day. After twenty days of this treatment, the tremors disappeared and never came back.

Case Y, May 1994

C. G. had been suffering from a nervous condition for over three months. She equipped a magnetic belt with nine 200-gauss magnets, south poles toward the skin, and wore the belt around her waist for one hour each morning and evening. She reported experiencing an amazing feeling of calm almost right away. Now, whenever she feels nervous or tired, C. G. applies the north pole of a 200-gauss magnet to her forehead, and her tension and fatigue disappear.

INFECTIONS

As previously indicated, one must be careful with magnetism in cases of infection. The south pole must never be applied to an infected area, as this pole stimulates growth and will only strengthen the infection. In cases of infection, only bipolar or north pole treatment should be used.

Case Z, October 1993

At thirty-eight years old, M. R. suffered from a persistent vaginal infection. She used a belt equipped with nine 200-gauss magnets, with the north poles against the skin, and wore it at night on her hips, about 7.5 cm under her navel. After six months of this treatment, the infection completely disappeared, and there has been no recurrence in two years.

Case AA, October 1995

K. F. suffered from a viral infection that attacked her nervous system, an illness known as Guillain-Barré syndrome. She experienced numbness in her wrists and was unable to lift anything or use her hands and feet. We had her hold the north pole of a large 1,500-gauss magnet in her hand, while her wrist was massaged with the south pole of an equal-strength magnet, and this treatment alternated from one hand/wrist to the other every ten minutes for a total of three hours. She underwent the same treatment again at home with the help of her family, and after three weeks of treatment, she was able to recover 30 percent of her hand mobility.

Her feet were also treated. A 1,500-gauss magnet was placed on the sole of her left foot, with the north pole against the skin, and another magnet of the same strength was applied to the sole of her right foot. This was done for twenty minutes, four times a day, and within two days her walking improved 70 to 80 percent.

TABLE 14. INFECTIONS

Case	Problem	Magnet	Pole	Duration	Observation
Z	Vaginal infection	Nine 200-gauss magnets	North	Overnight for six months	Infection disappeared and has not recurred after two years
AA	Viral infection: Guillain-Barré syndrome	Two 1,500-gauss magnets	North South	Massage three hours at a time	Regained 30% mobility after three weeks of treatment

MAGNETIZED WATER

As we saw in the previous chapter, magnetized water has positive effects on many different ailments. Our clients and friends have reported its many benefits, including relief from constipation, improved digestion, and better general health.

Case BB, February 1992

A. T. drinks six glasses of magnetized water a day and reports that she now has more energy at work.

Case CC, March 1992

H. I. drank six glasses of magnetized water a day for six months, and his chronic constipation disappeared completely.

Case DD, September 1992

At fifty-two, M. V. had been suffering from general exhaustion for eight years and had also experienced persistent numbness and cramps in her legs for over twelve years. She at first magnetized her water with twelve 1,500-gauss magnets, but she found that the water gave her severe headaches; so she reduced the number of magnets to three and then gradually increased them to six. After drinking a liter of this magnetized water per day for a month and a half, she reported that her energy had increased and she no longer had problems with her legs.

Case EE, April 1993

M. B. used magnetized water to treat a case of persistent diarrhea. She started to drink six to eight glasses a day, and after five days her stools became more consistent. Afterward she continued to drink magnetized water on a regular basis.

OTHER CASES

Case FF, March 1993

M. S. had a swollen tendon in her finger and consequently little flexibility. She rubbed the finger with the south pole of a 1,500-gauss magnet for fifteen minutes, and as a result the tendon relaxed and her finger regained flexibility. However, if she did not continue the treatment on a regular basis, the finger again became swollen.

Case GG, September 1995

A. G.'s toes were curled up from arthritis to such an extent that they did not touch the ground when she placed her feet on the floor, and her big toe protruded through the upper part of her shoe. In an effort to straighten out her toes, she applied six small 150-gauss magnets on each foot—three above the toes with the south pole against the skin and three under the toes with the north pole against the skin. She applied the magnets every night for three months, and after two months she experienced considerable improvement, though the condition was not completely cured.

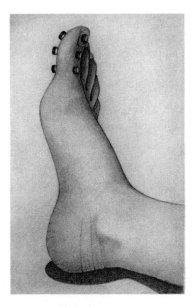

Fig. 37. Magnets on Toes

Case HH, August 1997

C. H. had a skin irritation on the palm of her left hand caused by a vegetable substance. When there was no improvement after two days, C. H. placed the north pole of a round, 2,000-gauss magnet on the palm and held it directly against the skin for two hours. The irritation disappeared completely, leaving only a small red circle about 1 cm in diameter, which took several more days to disappear. We now know what caused this local reaction: Being round, the magnet behaved like a ring-shaped magnet, the polarity of which is always inverted at the hole at the center. The polarity of the center of the round magnet was also reversed, and it was as though the south pole of a magnet had been applied to that particular spot. Given the properties of the south pole, it is not surprising that it produced a mild irritation.

CONCLUSION

We do not propose that magnet therapy should completely replace traditional medical treatment. However, we do suggest these two forms of treatment can be used in a complementary fashion. Magnet therapy can support and enhance traditional medical treatments. It can also sometimes provide relief when traditional medicine cannot.

We hope this book has awakened an interest in magnet therapy and convinced you of its many potential benefits. If you would like to further explore biomagnetism, there is a wealth of interesting literature available and ongoing research studies are published every year. Keep an open mind, but stay objective: Are the authors' theories plausible, and have they been confirmed by other studies? And if you read that a theory has not been "scientifically proven," does that mean it is untrue, or does it merely indicate that we do not yet have the tools and understanding necessary to prove it?

If you decide to conduct your own experiment on a particular biomagnetic phenomenon, make sure your methods are rigorous. Record your observations in full detail, including dates of treatment; the strength, type, and size of the magnets used; the pole used; placement of magnets (take pictures if necessary); exposure time; and treatment frequency. Try to determine as precisely as possible whether other factors might influence the outcome of your experiment, and discuss your observations with other people who use magnets therapeutically. Remember that an open but rigorous approach to learning is the best way to advance our knowledge in this field.

Also bear in mind that the characteristics and properties of magnetism described in this book are not necessarily the only ones. There is so much more to discover about this fascinating subject, and the conclusions we have presented here are not meant to be comprehensive or definitive. Our purpose is to disseminate as much information as possible about the benefits of magnet therapy and to encourage further interest and research. Although the benefits of magnetism cannot be disputed, more formal study and research are needed before it will be recognized by the scientific community.

It is our hope that the benefits of magnetism will one day be fully recognized and utilized by traditional medical professionals so that as many people as possible can experience its healing effects. But in the meantime, we urge you to take full advantage of the many benefits it offers.

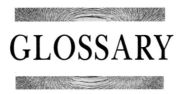

GLOSSARY

Biomagnetism: Applied science that studies the effects of magnetic energy on living organisms.

Curie point: The temperature above which ferromagnetic elements become paramagnetic (775°C for iron).

Diamagnetism: The property of materials in which the direction of induced magnetism is opposite to that of the induction field. This property describes all elements slightly repelled by a magnet.

Electromagnet: A device that produces a magnetic field, composed of two spools connected by a bar of soft iron through which an electric current passes.

Electromagnetic induction: The production of electric current in a circuit by varying the magnetic induction flow of the current.

Electromagnetism: A branch of physics that studies the interactions between electric currents and magnetic fields.

Ferrimagnetism: The magnetism found in ferrites. Ferrites are highly resistant materials with remarkable properties. They are used as transformer cores for high-frequency current, they are found in many types of electronic equipment, and they serve as memory components in computers.

Ferromagnetism: The property of materials with very high magnetic permeability (such as iron, nickel, cobalt), which retain residual magnetism in the absence of a magnetic field.

Galvanometer: Instrument used to measure low-intensity electric current.

Gauss: Unit of magnetic induction intensity produced by a magnetic pole and measured at 1 cm from that pole.

Induction lines: Representation of the magnetic energy in motion around a magnet.

Magnetic field: The area around a magnet in which its effects are felt.

Magnetic Field Deficiency Syndrome: Magnetic insufficiency characterized by various symptoms. The condition is difficult to diagnose because its symptoms are the same as those produced by hypertension, diabetes, or ataxia.

Magnetic pole: The point on the earth toward which the magnetic meridians converge. A magnet also has magnetic poles.

Magnetism: A branch of physics that studies the properties of magnets (natural or artificial) and associated phenomena.

Magnetite: The natural iron oxide Fe_3O_4, ferromagnetic black spinel (also called "magnet stone"), that is an excellent iron ore.

Magnetometer: Instrument used to measure and study variations in the earth's magnetic energy. Magnetometers used to measure factors such as declination, inclination, horizontal and vertical variants, and the total field are often called magnetic variometers. The instrument most frequently used to measure absolute declination is the magnetic theodolite. Generally the term "magnetometer" refers to any instrument used to measure the intensity of a magnetic field.

Magnetostriction: Phenomenon causing a substance to change volume when placed in a magnetic field. It occurs most obviously in the case of ferromagnetic materials.

Mesmerism: Eighteenth-century doctrine that held that all living beings are subject to the influence of a "magnetic fluid" that can be concentrated or rechanneled by "passes" and manipulation.

Oersted: Unit of magnetic induction intensity, measured in a vacuum.

Paramagnetism: The property of materials that, when exposed to a magnetic field, become magnetized in the same direction as iron, but much less intensely.

Polarity: Characteristic of a system having two poles.

Polarized: Having both poles; synonym of "magnetized."

Pole: Each of the extremities of a magnet or an electric circuit.

Solenoid: Elongated spool made of twisted conductor wire through which an electric current is passed. This creates a magnetic field inside the spool, which ceases to exist when the current is stopped.

FOR MORE INFORMATION

If you would like to receive additional information about magnet products or personal growth services please contact:

The Palmistry Center
c/o: Village Lac Dumouchel
576, Route 315
Chénéville, Québec
J0V 1E0
CANADA
Tel: (800) 307-2292 • (819) 428-4298
E-mail: mailbox@palmistry.com
Web site: www.palmistry.com

Heavenly Father, charge my body and my mind with Thy magnetism. And be Thou established in my soul, that I may be spiritually magnetic. By my love for Thee, I shall attract Thee unto me; and in Thee I shall have all things whatsoever I truly need. Aum . . . Amen*

Paramahansa Yogananda

---

*Paramahansa Yogananda, *The Divine Romance* (S.R.F., 1986), 140.

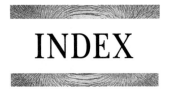

INDEX